WITHDRAWN

DISSIDENT
DOCTOR

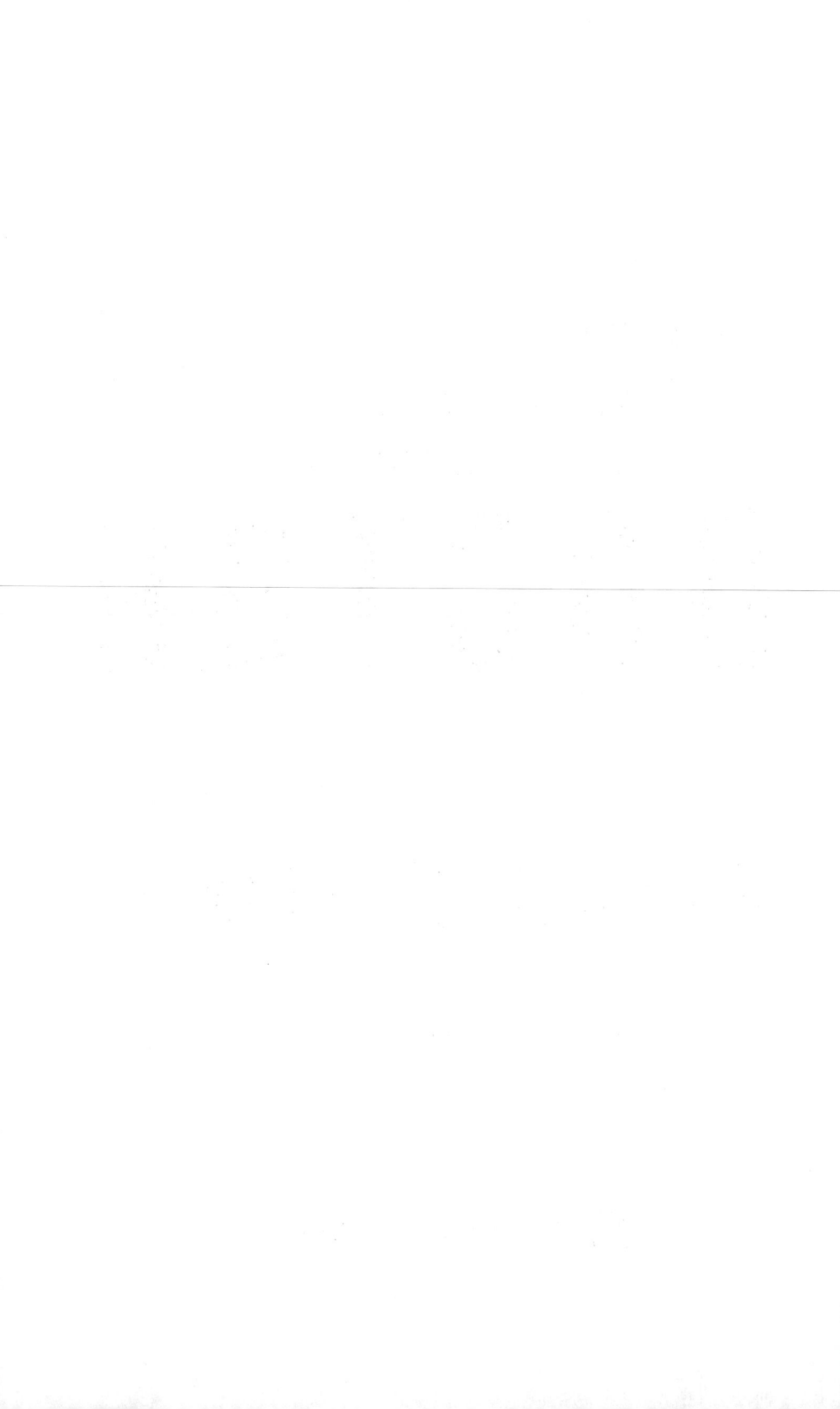

DISSIDENT

CATCHING BABIES AND CHALLENGING THE MEDICAL STATUS QUO

DOCTOR

MICHAEL C. KLEIN, MD

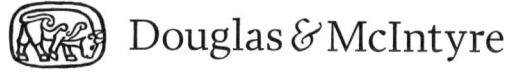 Douglas & McIntyre

Copyright © 2018 Michael C. Klein

1 2 3 4 5 — 22 21 20 19 18

All rights reserved. No part of this publication may be reproduced, stored in a retrieval system or transmitted, in any form or by any means, without prior permission of the publisher or, in the case of photocopying or other reprographic copying, a licence from Access Copyright, www.accesscopyright.ca, 1-800-893-5777, info@accesscopyright.ca.

Douglas and McIntyre (2013) Ltd.
P.O. Box 219, Madeira Park, BC, V0N 2H0
www.douglas-mcintyre.com

All photographs are from the author's collection except where otherwise noted.

The excerpt on pages 180–181 is reprinted from Michael C. Klein, "Too Close for Comfort? A Family Physician Questions Whether Medical Professionals Should Be Excluded from Their Loved Ones' Care," *Canadian Medical Association Journal*, January 1997, Volume 156, Issue 1, 53–55. © Canadian Medical Association 1997. This work is protected by copyright and the making of this copy was with the permission of the Canadian Medical Association Journal (www.cmaj.ca) and Access Copyright. Any alteration of its content or further copying in any form whatsoever is strictly prohibited unless otherwise permitted by law.

Edited by Amanda Lewis
Indexed by Emma Skagen
Dust jacket design by Anna Comfort O'Keeffe
Text design by Sari Naworynski

Printed and bound in Canada

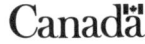 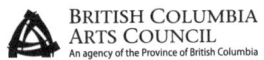

Douglas and McIntyre (2013) Ltd. acknowledges the support of the Canada Council for the Arts, which last year invested $153 million to bring the arts to Canadians throughout the country. We also gratefully acknowledge financial support from the Government of Canada and from the Province of British Columbia through the BC Arts Council and the Book Publishing Tax Credit.

Library and Archives Canada Cataloguing in Publication

Klein, Michael C., 1938-, author
    Dissident doctor : catching babies and challenging the medical status quo / Michael C. Klein.

Includes bibliographical references and index.
Issued in print and electronic formats.
ISBN 978-1-77162-192-2 (hardcover).--ISBN 978-1-77162-193-9 (HTML)

    1. Klein, Michael C., 1938-. 2. Physicians--Canada--Biography.
3. Midwifery--Canada. 4. Maternal health services--Canada. 5. Pediatrics--Canada. I. Title.

R464.K54A3 2018   610.92   C2018-902129-2
                                                  C2018-902130-6

To Dr. Howard Levy, who was jailed by the US Army for refusing to train Green Beret corpsmen, who would use their skills for political purposes. The other charge against him was "promoting disloyalty and disobedience" by discussing his anti-war views with GIs. Dr. Levy's treatment by the Army was central to my decision to try to avoid such an experience and, in the end, leave for Canada.

To my lawyer, John Somers, whose advice and advocacy (without his realizing it) prepared me to try to convince the US Army that I was more trouble than I was worth.

To our kids, Seth and Naomi, who put up with my rants at the dinner table, and with whom I partnered in helping with Bonnie's recovery. I am so proud of their values and contributions to making a better world. To Zoe, Toma and Aaron, our grandchildren, who light up our lives and who will carry the family story.

To my life partner, Bonnie, who despite her profound illness and disability, remains the force that holds our family together.

—◆—

TABLE OF CONTENTS

FOREWORD

MICHAEL KLEIN IS MY AGE, and because I have known him about half our lives, through tumultuous times in our world and in maternity care, my fascination with this book is deep. As I read it, I learned about this rugged individualist who thinks outside the box and can be very persuasive with his clear thinking and ability to support his beliefs with rational explanations and scientific evidence. The book enriched my knowledge of him and the interest we have shared for these many years—a passionate concern for the well-being of families from conception to successful, healthy integration of the family. For me, the book provided much background to explain how Michael came by his sense of justice, sharp wit and independent thinking skills that have led him to question widely accepted care practices that most clinicians follow without curiosity. Combine those traits with a feisty personality, a trace of stubbornness and a good deal of empathy for childbearing people, and you have a change-maker. I should add that Michael's analyses of published research are most helpful to those of us who lack the time or skills to objectively analyze and evaluate methods and conclusions of research studies. He is a good teacher.

Because I am what some call a "birth junkie," known for my work with doulas and childbirth education, I emphasize this area of our shared interest. This is not to minimize the importance of Michael's work in family practice, pediatrics, neonatology and the social determinants of health and the place of birth in the larger context of society's values. Michael's exposure to the

Red Scare and McCarthyism, his cross-cultural experiences in Mexico and Ethiopia, his struggles with the US Army and support for single-payer health care dating from his early years as a medical student at Stanford, and his own illnesses and the dramatic life-saving surgery for his wife, Bonnie (and his role in it)—all set the stage for his iconoclastic research on birth and critical analysis of old and new technologies. Michael thinks of himself not as a dispassionate physician-scientist but as a fully engaged human, free to use his own personal experiences within the therapeutic relationship.

Within family practice, his research emanates directly from questions posed by his patients or directly from his personal experience with family illness. As he puts it: "Apart from treating the condition, I could not afford *not* to look deeper into why the patient was vulnerable to the disease." Although a substantial portion of the book is about the challenges of providing high-quality caring birth environments for women and families, it is not a birth book. Michael uses birth as a window through which to understand the values of a society.

Because of my particular background and focus, I've decided to highlight several areas of maternity care where Michael has made unique and original contributions, thereby changing maternity care practices or raising questions that challenge current entrenched maternity care customs or "sacred cows." The bibliography at the end of the book includes references to his publications on these topics. I encourage readers to check out these sources. You will admire his critical-thinking skills and learn a lot! Although his studies are scientific, they are devoid of jargon and easy to read and understand by a general reader.

RESEARCH METHODOLOGY: CRITICAL EXAMINATION OF META-ANALYSES AND RANDOMIZED CONTROLLED TRIALS

Michael has authored numerous studies, commentaries and editorials analyzing and questioning the broad application of the findings of some meta-analyses (studies that group a number of research efforts together), demonstrating inconsistencies in which studies were or were not included and other flaws. Any of these flaws might skew the results. He has expressed these faults as "Garbage in; garbage out!" By carefully deconstructing the methodology and findings of many meta-analyses and systematic reviews, Michael has revealed fallacies in their design and conduct that led to reasonable doubts about their conclusions.

EPISIOTOMY

Some of Michael's early research questioned the value of liberal or routine use of episiotomy to prevent perineal lacerations or future pelvic floor relaxation. Although episiotomy was widely and unquestioningly practised for generations between 1921 through the 1980s, Michael asked if the purported advantages of episiotomy (prevention of tears, pelvic floor relaxation, urinary incontinence and postpartum pain, and improved later sexual functioning and pelvic floor strength) could be elucidated with a controlled trial. His landmark work, the only randomized controlled trial of episiotomy in North America, found that routine episiotomies caused the very trauma they were supposed to prevent. The best outcomes occurred in women not subjected to episiotomy across a wide range of outcomes.

After Michael's shocking findings were published, in the early 1990s, it took years before they were accepted widely. Indeed, there are still some practitioners who persist in performing episiotomies frequently or routinely. Michael's work, however, opened the door and has resulted in millions of women avoiding routine episiotomy and its harmful after-effects.

EPIDURAL ANALGESIA, BIRTH OUTCOMES AND DESIGN OF TRIALS

Michael and others have critically analyzed trials and meta-analyses comparing outcomes of labours with epidurals and without. They found that the conventional conclusions (most of which found no deleterious effects on outcomes, no increase in Caesarean rates nor difficulties breastfeeding, and others) were questionable because many critical variables were ignored or because the conditions of the trial did not approximate the way the technique was used in usual practice. Allowing such spurious research designs and findings to persist and disseminate makes critical evaluation of any technology difficult. Michael is fond of quoting his friend Phil Hall, who described many of the new "political" studies: "We have moved from evidence-based decision making to decision-based evidence making." In a related area, Michael investigated practice styles of various physicians and found that those whose patients had high epidural rates also had a style of practice that led to more fetal malpositions, more dysfunctional labours and higher intervention rates, all of which resulted in excess maternal/newborn morbidity.

ATTITUDES TOWARD BIRTH AND CORRESPONDING MANAGEMENT PRACTICES

Michael has long been curious about differences in attitudes toward maternity care in different subsets of birth workers and their relationship to differences in care practices. He has studied attitudes held by obstetricians—young versus old—family physicians, midwives, nurses and doulas, as well as childbearing women—demonstrating a relationship between providers' specialties or women's opinions about birth and their preferences for specific care practices, as well as differences by age of caregiver on birth plans, home birth, maternal informed choice and vaginal birth after a previous Caesarean. These studies of attitudes toward maternity care options may help inform efforts to align maternity care with the needs and wishes of childbearing families and encourage provision of understandable evidence-based information and support for parents' preferences.

Throughout his busy career, Michael has been an independent innovator—an early adopter of family-centred maternity care, midwifery in Canada and maternity care policies that foster parent-infant bonding, as well as a critic of Caesarean section on so-called maternal choice. He has been unusually supportive of "paraprofessionals" involved in maternity care, such as childbirth educators, doulas, lactation supporters and others. For us, he has been a much-needed and much-appreciated ally.

As you read this book, you will see the threads in his life that have shaped this "radical physician."

Penny Simkin, PT
Childbirth educator, doula trainer, lecturer
Author of *The Labor Progress Handbook, The Birth Partner, Pregnancy, Childbirth and the Newborn* and *When Survivors Give Birth*

INTRODUCTION

THIS IS MY STORY OF becoming a physician, and of how I followed a somewhat unorthodox path. I was a "red diaper baby," the child of left-wing parents. My early politicization and commitment to social justice influenced my decision to become a doctor and extended into my medical practice.

Some children grow into lefties like their parents, or they go in the opposite direction, becoming more like the dominant conservative culture. Many become politically cautious or apolitical as a defence against the hurt experienced by their parents and, by extension, themselves. Some never get over their anger against the system that stressed and damaged their family.

My parents were hounded during the McCarthy period and, even though they surrounded themselves with like-minded friends, were made to feel like the "other." Throughout high school and college, I too felt like an outsider because of my beliefs, which affected my relationships and my choice of medicine as a career and how I tried to integrate my beliefs into my future practice.

My education came not just from conventional medical school curricula but also from working as a medical student in different countries. I began practising medicine at a time when obstetrics was undergoing major changes, from often unjustified idiosyncratic practice to evidence-based practice, to the current era, when we are in a serious debate about the nature of evidence and the misuse of science for personal and political ends.

I transformed myself from a specialist in pediatrics and newborn intensive care to a family physician, the reverse of the usual, which is from generalist to specialist. I wholly embraced the new discipline of family medicine, which, beginning in the early 1970s, evolved from general practice into a holistic approach for individuals and their families. This profound change arose as a revolutionary response to over-specialized and impersonal care. As an academic discipline, the new family practice could take on the powerful specialties in a way that general practice couldn't.

I initially thought of obstetrics as a field better left to obstetricians and incompatible with office-based family practice, until I realized that maternity care, including attending births, could not only be done safely and well but is fundamental to community-based full-service family practice—what communities really need.

The patients' case histories illustrate the principle of *whole-person care* and the primacy of the individual in the context of the family and community. The famous Canadian physician and McGill medical graduate Sir William Osler wrote as much in *The Principles and Practice of Medicine* in 1892: "It is much more important to know what sort of a patient has a disease than what sort of a disease a patient has." Many of the patient stories illustrate the resilience of people and the strength of the human spirit. They demonstrate how innovative and unorthodox approaches can succeed in the face of difficult illnesses and experiences.

During the Vietnam War, when all physicians were drafted into the US medical military, I briefly became a military medical officer but avoided serving in that terrible war by fleeing to Canada with my wife, Bonnie. I am in the unusual position of having practised in Canada before the development of universal government-funded health care known in Canada as Medicare, then in the US without universal health care and finally, back in Canada when Medicare had been established. Having experienced the worst of US medical care, I decided to never again practise in the US. I fear today for Canadian health care as it drifts toward a US-style private model.

My story is also a love story. The deep relationship I share with my wife, Bonnie Sherr Klein, a filmmaker, author and disability activist, has shaped my life for more than fifty years. Bonnie's life-threatening illness more than thirty years ago highlighted my difficult and at times controversial role in advocating for her care or reluctantly providing some of her care as a husband

and physician. Bonnie's illness and prolonged recovery changed our family, my practice and me. I wasn't exposed to so-called alternative therapies in medical school and was therefore skeptical, but through Bonnie's illness and my own back pain, I finally came to understand how "soft" methods could be successfully integrated into practice.

Because of my background as a pediatric and newborn care specialist, it was logical for me to became a practitioner and researcher in maternity and newborn care, thereby bridging the disciplines of obstetrics and gynecology, pediatrics, family practice and midwifery. Contesting conventional wisdom for unjustified procedures, such as routine use of episiotomy and Caesarean section on demand, shaped the way I practised and how I used research to alter practice for myself and others.

By focusing on the needs of pregnant women and families rather than the needs of medical practitioners, I connected with midwifery at a time when it was not yet legal in Canada. With others, I worked to see midwifery legalized and regulated in an era when a physician working with midwives was so unfathomable that I was ostracized by some of my family physician colleagues.

Although birth, in the form of birth stories, research and politics, comprises an important part of this book, this is not a birth book. I use birth as a metaphor, a window into health care and our values as a society. My joy and awe in assisting at birth was often the stimulus if not the cure for my practice as a family physician caring for patients whose lives were often sad or who were suffering from incurable diseases.

Throughout my career, I worked not as an impersonal physician-scientist but as a human using my own experiences with health and illness as the bedrock of how I see normal medical care. I tried to practise medicine in an ethical and humane way, despite the many forces that make such practice increasingly difficult.

"It is much more important to know what sort of a patient has a disease than what sort of a disease a patient has."
—Sir William Osler (1849–1919)

1. A BUNCH OF LEFTIES

THERE WERE NO DOCTORS IN my family. My parents were born into poor families in Newark, New Jersey. My paternal grandfather was a tailor who became blind from untreated diabetes. My mother, Annie, was the youngest in her family and very close to her brother, Harold, who tried to protect her from restrictions placed on her by their traditional "Old World" parents, who aspired for her to work only as a salesgirl. She did so but was ultimately fired for her union organizing. Her father was a bus owner/driver, bought out by a large public service bus company. He later worked with his brother-in-law as a fishmonger. Annie's two sisters, Betty and Sarah, lived a conventional life. Betty worked in a small neighbourhood grocery store that she owned with her husband, Ychiel.

The next-to-youngest of six siblings, my father, Philip, went to art school but was distracted by extensive left-wing political activities. He was finally expelled, with this admonition in his letter of dismissal: "You are a great artist. If you get serious and drop outside activities, you will go far."

In the early days of the civil war in Spain, the Nazis had developed a cozy relationship with fascist Franco, who was trying to defeat the anti-fascist Loyalists in order to establish a fascist state in Spain. The Loyalists appealed for international support to defeat Franco, and a number of our family friends joined the Abraham Lincoln Brigade and went to Spain to fight. Many on the left recognized that this battle was the beginning of a wider war not just in Europe but for the hearts and souls of the civilized world. Some of our friends died in that war, and the stories of their doomed sacrifice were legendary in our family.

During the Spanish Civil War, my parents met at the Jack London Club, a left-wing gathering place for disaffected young folks. Annie's brother, Harold, recruited her to the club. They were all products of the Depression and hoped for a better world, and they acted politically on their beliefs. One of my father's older brothers, Sol, was so disaffected with society and the government of the day that after graduating from architecture school in the US and unable to find a job, as nothing was being built during the Depression, he moved with his wife, Pauline, to the Soviet Union—ironically, perhaps, since by being born in Newark, Sol had not endured the Russian pogroms that his parents had escaped by moving to the US. Sol's two children, about my age, were both born in Moscow. Eva became a physician and Joseph an engineer. Throughout World War II, Sol designed oil refineries at a secret site in the city of Ufa in the Ural Mountains.

Uncle Sol and his family lived in Moscow among other North American expatriates, most of whom were Jewish. These transplanted Americans lived, and many still do, in the same dreary multi-storey building, where most spoke English and maintained an isolated "American" mini-society. My cousin Joseph married Vicki, the child of New York Jews. I always got a kick out of the fact that Vicki taught English to generations of unsuspecting Muscovites, who failed to realize they were learning to speak English with a Brooklyn accent.

In the era of the "refuseniks," many Russian Jews declared their support for Israel and finally expressed their ethnicity and even their desire to emigrate to Israel. Before this time, my Russian family and their neighbours denied their Jewishness. They claimed to be thoroughly integrated into Soviet life, yet all their friends and neighbours were Jewish. When I visited in the early 1980s, I asked to see the famous Moscow synagogue. My cousins claimed not to know where it was. Later, one of their children immigrated to Israel and moved to a settlement on the West Bank, next door to Avigdor Lieberman, one of the most right-wing members of the Israeli cabinet, who in 2016 became minister of defence. He believes in a one-state solution—expulsion of the Palestinians.

Philip's oldest brother, David, was a plumber who wanted to be a doctor. As my grandparents were much older when my father was born, David served in the parental role. My father's brother Issie was an artist, animator and role model for my father. As I. Klein, he published about two hundred cartoons and drawings in the *New Yorker* between the late 1920s and 1930s.

Brother Daniel was the intellectual of the family, who received his PhD in pharmacology and worked for drug companies in various capacities. Sister Lillian was the baby and doted on by all the brothers. She married a rather unpleasant, very religious man, who abused her psychologically, while unsuccessfully trying to convert the rest of the family to his religious proclivities.

My parents' union and left-wing political activities set the stage for the next four decades of their life and, by extension, mine. In the late 1930s, having left-wing values was not unusual. But despite being allies in World War II, the Soviet Union's path became increasingly worrisome to US leadership. The early left-wing political experiences of my parents and many others created serious problems for them in the McCarthy period of the 1950s to the end of the Vietnam War era and beyond.

2. WALT DISNEY SHAPES EVERYTHING

I WAS BORN IN CALIFORNIA in 1938 while my dad was working as an animator for Walt Disney. His brother Issie had recruited him to go west. Issie had worked on *Popeye* and *Little Lulu*. He taught my dad animation and arranged for his Disney job. My dad's first contract with Disney was for twenty-four dollars per week and contained a clause prohibiting him from working for other studios for two years after leaving Disney—a controlling characteristic that shaped his hatred for Walt Disney for the rest of his life.

My younger brother, Henry, inherited the family artistic skill. He worked as a graphic artist, printmaker and teacher in several places before settling in Los Angeles, where he taught graphic art for many years in a community college. He also used his art to protest the Vietnam War. In his retirement, he represents many graphic artists from the former Soviet bloc. Before the fall of the Soviet Union, the artists he represented used, and still use, their art to contest their political establishments. Anti-Stalin, anti-Soviet and now anti-authoritarian political messages are often buried in their prints.

In near poverty, my parents paid for my mother's prenatal care and my birth by giving the doctor animation cells of Donald Duck and other Disney characters. The family lore paints this doctor as a kind of Robin Hood character. "Don't worry about the money," the doctor was to have said. "Let the starlets pay for it." Many years later, my dad inexplicably gave away all of his original cartoon cells to a stranger who claimed to be opening a museum of animation. They would have been hugely valuable today.

My mother's Caesarean section was undertaken without charge because she had a "tipped womb" and was "too small" for a vaginal birth. A "tipped womb" is a womb that is pointed to the back, rather than in its usual place, flexed forward. A tipped womb is irrelevant to the success of delivering vaginally, since as the pregnancy progresses, the womb moves in the only direction it can, straight upward. Caesarean section rates in 1938 were about 3 per cent, compared to well over 25 per cent today. In gratitude, my mother often told the story of her wonderful and very generous doctor.

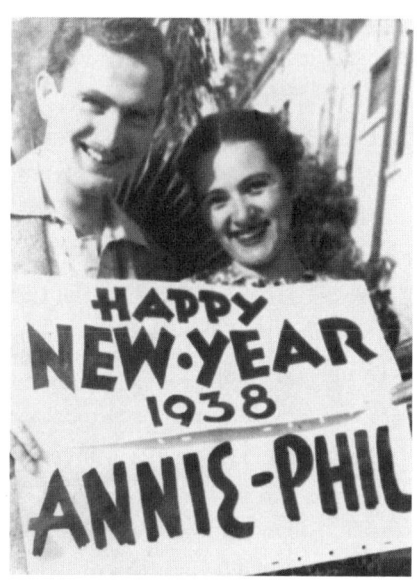

My parents, Annie and Philip Klein, in 1938. My mom is pregnant with me.

The dictum of the day was "once a section, always a section." Since I was born by Caesarean, in which the doctor employed the then-conventional large vertical abdominal incision, my brother was also born four years later by Caesarean, my mom receiving another large vertical incision and resultant scar. When I was about twelve years old, I accompanied my mother to a Newark hospital where she received radiation treatment for a large, thick and painful vertical Caesarean scar. This type of vertical incision is not done today, nor is radiotherapy for this purpose. Almost certainly because of her radiation therapy for her Caesarean scar, when my mother was in her eighties she had urgent surgery for a huge abdominal aneurism, large enough to be in danger of rupturing and possibly killing her. The aneurism was located directly below the zone of her radiotherapy treatment from the two Caesareans, the first of which she should probably never have had in the first place.

Out of the blue, at my parents' fiftieth anniversary, my mom brought forth a book that contained all her prenatal care records and her prenatal X-ray results, which were apparently the basis for the doctor declaring that she was too small to deliver vaginally. We do not take pelvic X-rays these days, as they produce too much radiation, and the only way to know if a woman is really too small is to have her try to give birth vaginally. Surprisingly, small woman can deliver large babies, whereas large women may have difficulties delivering vaginally. We just don't know which women will deliver vaginally, and most predictions are wrong.

Faced with the bonanza of my mom's prenatal records, I could not resist studying her actual listed internal dimensions taken from the X-rays. As modern obstetrics textbooks do not even present the X-ray pelvic dimensions for use as a management tool, I had to look up the normal values for X-ray pelvic internal dimensions in my 1950 edition of the most commonly used obstetric textbook of the day. This allowed me to compare my mom's listed internal dimensions with normal values. Her pelvis was *enormous*! So I really can't know what the motivation was for my mom to have a pre-emptive Caesarean.

I decided not to share my investigation with my mother, as to do so would only make her feel bad and spoil a good family story. I later became aware of the cascade of adverse events unleashed by her first Caesarean delivery, but at the time I had not yet committed to the maternity care research and practice that was to characterize so many of my future endeavours. Some have said that my own Caesarean birth, and the consequences for my mother, set me on a path that continues to this day, in which I look deeply at old and new technologies in birth and study their effectiveness or lack thereof. And they might be right. Or not.

Slaving away for Disney in the late 1930s, well before the era of computer animation, my dad spent six months working on a single scene in the belly of the whale in *Pinocchio* (twenty-five frames per second—all drawn by hand). While working on *Fantasia, Snow White and the Seven Dwarfs, Bambi* and *Pinocchio*, my dad was also one of the key union organizers of the Screen Cartoonists Guild. In 1941, during the famous five-month strike designed to unionize Disney, we lived in a tent on a lot across the road from the Burbank Disney Studios, cooking over open fires. I am told that every morning I would sit on somebody's motorcycle and scream in a high-pitched voice, "Scab!" when strikebreakers went through the studio gates. My political training started early.

At the age of three, because my parents were so engaged with the strike, I was sent to a farm where the owners supported the strikers. My memory of being able to sit on the tractors and pet the farm animals is still strong, but I also remember crying from missing my parents. My parents' Los Angeles home was a refuge for many activists. After coming to California from Oklahoma, Woody Guthrie stayed at our house for a while. Our house was also the site for meetings of those who sought to change the way that workers at Disney were treated.

When the strike at Disney was finally settled and the union was established, the union organizers were dismissed. My dad's notice from Disney reads: "It is necessary to reduce our staff and we are sorry to have to extend your present layoff indefinitely." With the war effort in full swing, my dad went to work in the shipyards of Los Angeles, where he learned a new skill as a welder of Liberty ships.

The "incompetent" and "redundant" union organizers moved back east, where several of them established new studios like United Productions of America (UPA), first making army training films to support the war effort and later *The Nearsighted Mr. Magoo, Gerald McBoing-Boing* and *Dick Tracy*. Joseph McCarthy's House Un-American Activities Committee (HUAC) later branded UPA communist influenced.

When I was four, we moved back from Los Angeles to the family home in Newark, where my brother, Henry, was born. My dad continued to be a welder on Liberty ships, then based in shipyards in Hoboken, across the Hudson River from New York City. These ships ran the dangerous North Atlantic gauntlet to supply Europe with the needed arms and supplies to defeat the Nazis. When my dad was welding keels deep in the holds of the ships, there was no ear protection from the extreme noise nor breathing protection from the various pollutants—leading ultimately to my dad's severe cardiac and lung disease, abetted by forty years of smoking. I have a special engraved hammer, awarded to my dad for having welded "the straightest keel." I remember my dad leaving for work in early mornings when it was still dark, returning late at night, exhausted and not available for play. My mother filled the parental gap, seeing to our educational and recreational needs, often taking my brother and me to museums and cultural events and reading with us on a regular basis.

Somehow the army found out that my dad was a film animator working in the shipyards, and they felt that he could better contribute to the war effort as an animator. They threatened to draft him to make army training films if he refused to be reassigned. In a photograph of his production unit on the roof of a New York City studio, he is the only civilian in the Signal Corps, the army film unit.

Post-war, my father was employed in animation in New York in the early days of television. Life seemed to settle down. Work in this new medium kept him busy, animating dancing cigarettes for Lucky Strike, as well as doing technical animation, explaining how various machines worked. Again, he would commute by bus or train very early in the morning from Newark to Manhattan, returning exhausted well after dark. It was not until years later that I came to appreciate his sacrifice to keep the family solvent.

Whereas my mother was very positive and funny, my dad was tired and remote and went to bed early. He tried to read to us but often fell asleep in the middle of the story. My mother helped me with my homework, acted as a sounding board for my ideas and attended my swimming meets. Unfortunately, she was unable to help me with my increasing difficulties with math. I attribute these difficulties to the punitive style of one teacher, to whose room I seemed to be regularly assigned throughout grammar school. Could be that I am just lousy at math.

3. WOCHICA

THROUGHOUT THE RUN-UP TO WORLD WAR II, my mom sent letters from California to her family back in New Jersey in which she extolled the virtues of the Soviet Union, where everyone was treated equally. Like many lefties of their generation, my parents thought that the Soviet Union would be the answer to the inequality and degradation experienced by workers worldwide, and that she experienced coming from a poor working-class family, as did my father. My mom somehow managed to rationalize the pact between the Soviet Union and Germany—even when information was leaking out about the treatment of Jews in Germany, Eastern Europe and later the Soviet Union. In the end, when it became impossible to deny the truth of Stalin's behaviour toward Jews and other dissenters, my parents finally became disillusioned with the actions of the Soviet Union, and the letters changed in tone and content.

Despite their disenchantment with the Soviet Union, my parents held on to their core values of racial and social equality. Post-war, I remember being taken to Paul Robeson concerts in Newark and being sent to an interracial summer camp called WOCHICA. I always thought WOCHICA was a Native American name. Turns out that it stood for Workers' Children's Camp. That first summer, at seven, I was the youngest child in the bunk and missed my parents. The next summer at age eight, I was no longer lonely. The camp was formative. I grew up singing folk songs about justice and racial equality, a very different experience from my grammar and later high school classmates, so much so that I kept my progressive ideas to myself. Very early, I knew that ours were different from the dominant culture's values and beliefs.

The singing at WOCHICA was a huge part of the camp experience, including songs about China's Long March against the nationalists under Chiang Kai-shek, which led to the founding of modern Mainland China under Mao Zedong. Paul Robeson was a regular visitor at the camp, as well as Pete Seeger and other progressive artists. The main hall at the camp was actually named Paul Robeson Hall. I have an indelible memory of, at the age of eight, hearing Robeson sing at noon and learning to swim that very afternoon. The Ku Klux Klan eventually closed down WOCHICA during the McCarthy period, burning a cross on the camp lawn. As the Red Scare infected the country and US politics moved further to the right, the camp managers became fearful for the safety of the children and reluctantly decided to close the camp.

My parents consistently supported progressive causes. In 1948, when I was ten, my parents worked for the Progressive Party and Henry Wallace in his unsuccessful bid for the presidency of the United States against Harry Truman. My brother and I accompanied my parents on various marches, demonstrations and political rallies, even taking the train to Washington to protest in front of the White House against the planned execution of the Rosenbergs as presumptive atomic spies. I was too young to really know what I was protesting, but along I went.

Our secret "different" beliefs were not so completely secret. Some of my grammar school and high school classmates still remember that I called my parents by their given names, Anne and Phil, rather than Mom and Dad—unheard of. It was something our parents taught us, an expression of egalitarianism.

As a preteen, I would take the bus to New York to visit various museums and often meet my dad for lunch at his studio, where he would show me his work and introduce me to his co-workers. One of them was Leon Bibb, a Black singer-actor who supported his singing and acting career by working in animation. In the 1950s, Leon was blacklisted for his "radical" beliefs and activities—among them his support of Robeson, who became a godfather to one of his children. Leon was a friend and colleague of Paul Robeson,

Sidney Poitier and Harry Belafonte. In the 1960s, he had a successful series of appearances on *The Ed Sullivan Show*, and when I was in high school, I saw Leon perform in a New York theatre in *A Hand Is on the Gate*, the first all-Black musical, featuring James Earl Jones, Ruby Dee and many other stunning singers and actors. In a strange turn of fate, when Bonnie and I moved to Vancouver in 1993, we found that Leon had also moved there and had purchased a condo across the hall from us. He became our dear friend. In 2016, when Leon became seriously ill and confined to a nursing home, Bonnie and I continued to visit him. A day before he died, I had the pleasure of sitting beside him during our daughter Naomi's and her husband Avi's Vancouver film opening of *This Changes Everything*. Although he was blind, the film audio told enough of the story for Leon to be fully engaged, commenting and exhorting throughout.

When I was twelve, on one of my regular excursions to New York, one painting in particular had a profound effect on me. At the Museum of Modern Art, I saw Picasso's famous *Guernica*, depicting the bombing in 1937 of that Spanish city. The Nazis were testing out their planes and their developing war machine on anti-fascist Loyalists, killing hundreds of women and children.

When I think about the independence of taking the bus alone to New York and wandering around unsupervised in museums, I am struck by how parents today keep their children under much closer control. I don't remember being afraid to travel alone or worried about my safety. Obviously, my parents were not worried either.

4. MY JEWISH EDUCATION

ALTHOUGH MY PARENTS SPOKE ENGLISH, they also spoke Yiddish, the language of their family homes. They were cultural, not religious, Jews but did not deny their Jewish heritage, connecting with Jewish left-wing history. Yiddish was the language of the working-class Jews, who lived in a parallel society in Newark, Brooklyn and the Lower East Side of New York City. My parents thought that learning Hebrew, the new spoken language of Israel, was contrived. Nevertheless, we understood the place of Hebrew as a means of distinguishing the new Israelis from their Yiddish-speaking Eastern European roots and the Holocaust.

For my parents, it made sense to enroll me in a Yiddish folk school, rather than the schools where my friends and classmates were studying Hebrew in preparation for their bar mitzvahs. I did not last long in the Yiddish folk school. On the way to class with my Yiddish books, some gentile kids beat me up and threw my books down a sewer. When I arrived late and told the rather stiff and punitive teacher the story of the attack, he dismissed it as a fabrication. When I needed comfort and understanding, he called me a liar. I refused to return to the school. My Jewish education was over.

Although I was acutely aware of being different, I cannot remember objecting to the path that my parents had selected for me. While my Jewish classmates were preparing for their bar mitzvahs, I was often alone. I used my time to study clarinet and perfect my swimming skills. For my mom and many other Jews, clarinetist Benny Goodman was an iconic figure. As a Jewish role model in the big band and jazz era, what could be better? Maybe the violin. To make ends meet, my clarinet teacher, Charlie Anderson, played clarinet at the Empire Burlesque in Newark. He was a gentle and supportive teacher who taught me up to a point and then transferred my music education to an older bandleader who had his own community orchestra. It was in that setting that I perfected my ability to play in musical groups of various sizes.

The devotion to swimming and clarinet were positive benefits of being separate from my peers at a formative time. As an attempt to fit in, for a few months I even attended Young Pioneer activities that were designed to turn us on to Israel and entice us to travel there to work on a kibbutz. Although I did not intend to immigrate to Israel, I liked to drive tractors in the country, and the girls were great.

5. THE RED SCARE

BECAUSE WE NEEDED A PLACE where our family felt at home, we built a summer house by hand in northern New Jersey, close to other like-minded families. We worked on it during summers and weekends over many years. My dad, my mom and us kids cleared the land. We split rocks, dug out stumps and learned some carpentry. Eventually, my father was unemployable because of his political history, so he funnelled his creative energies into that wonderful family home, near a camp that had been built by anti-Nazi Germans who fled during the rise of Hitler. It was called Camp Midvale and was run initially by Nature Friends of America, which eventually found itself on the US Attorney General's list of supposedly subversive organizations.

It was an interracial camp, which I never thought was unusual. Like at WOCHICA, regular entertainers included Pete Seeger and the Weavers, Paul Robeson and other progressives. Camp Midvale was where I finally developed comfortable friendships with other "red diaper babies," boys and girls with whom I could openly share values and beliefs. On weekends, the camp often hosted Black people from Paterson, New Jersey, who because of segregation had been prohibited from swimming in a public pool. And this was northern

New Jersey! One Sunday, working as a camp lifeguard, I recall rescuing a half-dozen Black men who were in deep water for the first time in their lives.

In a strange repetition of the WOCHICA event, the Klan burned a cross on the camp's lawn. The Klan also torched the recreation hall and effectively closed down the camp. Local police were not perturbed. The fire department did not bother to come, and the police did nothing to investigate the perpetrators. It was at the height of the McCarthy period, and I am sure that conventional governmental sources were pleased to see the camp closed. It was a frightening time. In 1949, I vividly remember friends returning to the camp from an event in Peekskill, New York, where a civil rights concert featuring Paul Robeson had taken place. Attendees leaving the concert had to run a police-organized gauntlet of screaming mobs who lined their only escape route. While the New York State Police stood by, the mob pelted the cars and buses of attendees with rocks. Hundreds were injured. As an eleven-year-old, the event imprinted on my memory the consequences of having different beliefs and values.

Over many decades and after several iterations, the New Jersey Audubon Society finally bought the camp and turned it over to a local nature group in perpetuity. It has maintained its incredible outdoor swimming pool fed by a natural waterfall, the place where I honed my competitive swimming skills, worked as a lifeguard and swimming instructor, and received my Red Cross instructor certificate at a much younger age than was legitimate. That certificate opened doors to several jobs. Our son, Seth, also worked as a lifeguard at the camp, where he too began his education in social justice.

My work at Camp Midvale, and later my work at country clubs, exposed me to new friends and work colleagues and led to a competitive swimming career and college swimming scholarship. It also resulted in leadership roles that probably set me up to be chair or director of several departments of family practice in later years.

In the 1950s, the Red Scare was part of our everyday lives. On one occasion, two of my friends and their mother were staying at Camp Midvale. The mother and children were family of a known communist leader who was in hiding to prevent arrest. Every day in the camp parking lot sat a Ford Falcon containing two FBI agents. We knew they were FBI agents because we three boys approached the car and asked them who they were and they confirmed their identity. The family had been followed wherever they went, the idea being that their fugitive communist father would probably try to contact his family and be arrested when he did.

One hot day in the summer, we decided to have some fun. We planned a long overnight hike high in the adjacent forest. Outfitted in camping clothes, and with lots of food and supplies, we ostentatiously passed the FBI agents in the parking lot and set out for the mountains. As we knew they would, the FBI agents quickly disembarked and began following us in their suits, ties and city shoes. We hiked high in the mountains and after several hours made camp, pitched our tent and began cooking dinner. Of course the agents had no food, water or shelter. We could easily see them down the trail sitting on the ground. The cooking smells must have been terrible for them, but that was the idea. The next day we retraced our steps and came abreast of the agents, deliberately emptying our canteens on the ground. It was a satisfying trip, particularly for the children of the fugitive.

During World War II and the early part of the Korean War, making army training films within the Signal Corps in New York City was patriotic. But during the height of the McCarthy era, my father's early life as a left-wing union organizer came back to haunt him. My father's boss in New York valued his work, so he at first made my father's personnel file disappear during security sweeps, but in the end the company found this too risky and laid my father off.

Because of his early union activities and the exploding Red Scare, my father assumed that he would be brought before the infamous House Un-American Activities Committee (HUAC). Many of our family friends had been before the committee, along with Pete Seeger and other so-called fellow travellers. The purpose of the HUAC was to intimidate and get reluctant witnesses to name names, to protect their own personal safety. Refusing would have led to contempt of Congress and imprisonment. Many witnesses did name names, and people who we considered our friends named my father and close family friends. Some of those who broke down did so out of abject fear for themselves and their families. I remember being coached on how to behave if the FBI came calling. We expected a knock on the door, which never came.

Blacklisted, my father was forced to work at home under a pseudonym, making obscure cartoons and comic books. His drafting table was placed in the middle of the living room in our small Newark apartment. It was impossible not to feel my dad's tension and frustration with this hated and demeaning work. It was worse for some of my friends, whose fathers went into hiding. To keep himself amused, my dad often inserted members of our extended family into the cartoons—an aunt who was a buffoon would appear as a buffoon; an uncle who was mean and insincere would appear as such. Although I wasn't sure exactly why, I certainly got the message that one or both of my parents could be taken away and jailed for their beliefs and activities. This experience deeply scarred some of my contemporaries, whose parents were named in the McCarthy witch hunts. Some became lefties, but most retreated into an apolitical and fearful life, whereas others never got over their anger at being forced to hide or dissemble, expressing their history through distrust and perpetual feelings of alienation.

Because my dad could not work during the McCarthy period, my mother was forced to take over as the breadwinner. Her father would have been surprised to see how independent and skilled she became. When I went away to Oberlin College, to make ends meet, and prepare for the next phase of her life, my mother went to Rutgers University as a classmate of the very girls with whom I had graduated high school. They appreciated her as a kind of mother figure, and she was wonderfully successful in college and graduate school. She ultimately became a much sought-after special education and reading specialist from the 1960s onward.

The McCarthy period led to mass firings of anyone suspected of left-wing leanings. The Hollywood Ten, including Dalton Trumbo, the famous Hollywood screenwriter, were blacklisted and wrote under pen names. Closer to home, the head of the language department at my high school lost his job. For many years, to get by he had to sell insurance, until he was finally exonerated and received fifteen years of back pay.

The late Pete Seeger's 1955 testimony before the HUAC, excerpted here, is a milestone in defiance and ought to be read by anyone who loves democracy and personal integrity. Although he was not indicted, he tied the committee up in knots and made them look like the hateful, mean-spirited publicity seekers that they were.

Mr. SEEGER: I am not going to answer any questions as to my association, my philosophical or religious beliefs or my political beliefs, or how I voted in any election, or any of these private affairs. I think these are very improper questions for any American to be asked, especially under such compulsion as this. I would be very glad to tell you my life if you want to hear of it...

I feel that in my whole life I have never done anything of any conspiratorial nature and I resent very much and very deeply the implication of being called before this Committee that in some way because my opinions may be different from yours, or yours, Mr. Willis, or yours, Mr. Scherer, that I am any less of an American than anybody else. I love my country very deeply, sir.

Mr. TAVENNER: You said that you would tell us about the songs. Did you participate in a program at Wingdale Lodge in the State of New York, which is a summer camp for adults and children, on the weekend of July Fourth of this year?

Mr. SEEGER: Again, I say I will be glad to tell what songs I have ever sung, because singing is my business... But I decline to say who has ever listened to them, who has written them, or other people who have sung them.

Mr. TAVENNER: Did you sing this song, to which we have referred, "Now Is the Time," at Wingdale Lodge on the weekend of July Fourth?

Mr. SEEGER: I don't know any song by that name, and I know a song with a similar name. It is called "Wasn't That a Time." Is that the song?

Chairman WALTER: Did you sing that song?

Mr. SEEGER: I can sing it. I don't know how well I can do it without my banjo.

Chairman WALTER: I said, did you sing it on that occasion?

Mr. SEEGER: I have sung that song. I am not going to go into where I have sung it. I have sung it many places.

Chairman WALTER: Did you sing it on this particular occasion? That is what you are being asked.

Mr. SEEGER: Again my answer is the same... I will tell you about the songs, but I am not going to tell you or try to explain—

Chairman WALTER: I direct you to answer the question. Did you sing this particular song on the Fourth of July at Wingdale Lodge in New York?

Mr. SEEGER: I have already given you my answer to that question, and all questions such as that. I feel that is improper: to ask about my associations and opinions. I have said that I would be voluntarily glad to tell you about any song, or what I have done in my life.

Although Seeger's "performance" before the committee was memorable, that committee meeting was also the beginning of Seeger's inability to work. The Weavers were Seeger's main singing group. Despite their earlier considerable success on radio, TV, and in clubs and concerts, bookings dried up. He and the Weavers survived by singing on the college circuit to great appreciation. In fact, it was the beginning of the folk revival: "Goodnight, Irene," "If I Had a Hammer," "Where Have All the Flowers Gone?"

The final demise of McCarthy, and for a time McCarthyism, began with a famous program by Edward R. Murrow, a much-beloved newscaster, who devoted a full program to detailing the damages to the US caused with the wave of McCarthyism. Murrow's impact was detailed in the 2005 film *Good Night, and Good Luck*, starring George Clooney.

In 1956, just after I left for Oberlin College, my parents moved permanently to their home near Camp Midvale. Here they could finally live among friends who shared their values and political beliefs. My last act before leaving for college was to dig a cellar by hand. Because I hit bedrock at five feet, it became a split-level home. I still have the calluses of the dig, acquired because the family did not want to sacrifice any trees, which would have happened if we had used a backhoe to do the excavation.

When my dad was finally forcibly retired, he turned to his first love—painting—but he was frustrated, as all of his early output looked like Disney. Thankfully, his welding skills allowed him to escape Disney by turning to metal sculpture. His many sculptures adorn our house and grounds on the Sunshine Coast near Vancouver, British Columbia, though the early metal sculptures do have the look of *Fantasia*.

6. IMPLICATIONS OF MY EARLY HISTORY

IN HIGH SCHOOL, THE TENSION of being different and at risk of discovery was ever present. I attended Weequahic High School, a school with a large Jewish population, which was attended by Jerry Lewis and Philip Roth and was the setting for Roth's early novels. To my friends and classmates, I was just one of the guys, captain of the swimming team and first clarinet in the orchestra and band. I dated some young women in my class, but as we didn't share values, these relationships were superficial and short-lived. On rare occasions, I was able to date a few "red diaper babies," who generally came from New York City.

I got my driver's licence early, and my parents often let me take the family car. I regularly ferried my teammates to swimming practice. But when I would drive our car through Black neighbourhoods on the way to swim practice or swim meets, my teammates would occasionally shout racial epithets out the car window. Unwilling to go into detail about my beliefs, which clearly clashed with theirs, all I could do was tell them that if they continued they would have to walk. They couldn't understand what was up with me. "What's your problem? You like niggers?" The practice pool was located in the very area that later became the epicentre of the infamous 1967 Newark riots, where large numbers of angry Black youths burned down huge areas of the "ghetto."

Before and during high school, I worked in my uncle Harold's furniture factory, the same uncle who introduced my mother to left-wing activities. The factory was located a short walk from the practice pool in the Black area that was later torched. Uncle Harold had excellent relationships in the Black neighbourhood, so when the riots took place, his factory was one of the few businesses spared the torch. I was given a large degree of responsibility in managing the facility in the evenings, even selling some furniture. Typically, I would walk down to the factory showroom after swimming practice, have dinner at a local diner, and then start my shift at the factory, doing my homework until customers arrived.

Despite my double life, I loved high school. I had some wonderful teachers, but my deficiency in math continued from my grammar school days. I only got as far as trigonometry—with great difficulty. This was made up for by success in other studies. I loved history and was taught writing and analytical skills by Mrs. Sadie Raus, whose support and encouragement were to prove very important in my future endeavours.

For a young person, being the "other" is inevitably traumatic. Teenagers usually want to be like everyone else. Compensation also can express itself through the need to excel, to overcome being "different" by striving to be the best. This in turn can lead to an arrogance that in my case might be seen as a personality flaw.

I volunteered as a swimming instructor at the Kessler Institute in northern New Jersey, a role that was instrumental in my eventual application to medical school. It was a rehabilitation facility run by the United Mine Workers union for members who had spinal injuries from mining accidents. Most were paraplegics. I was impressed by the physiotherapists, under whose professional control I worked. I so appreciated their work that I planned to be one. Soon, however, I realized that the physiotherapists got their orders from orthopaedic surgeons, so I began to think about being an orthopaedic surgeon.

I was attracted to medicine, in part, from the family experience of being at risk because of political ideas. This followed directly from my father being expelled from art school for his political ideas, fired by Disney for union organizing and red-baited from his job as an animator during the McCarthy period. Looking at my career options, I was attracted to what I perceived as the independence afforded by medicine. Medicine would protect me from unpredictable organizational or business politics. I had the idea that as a physician

I would not be dependent on anyone else. In part, this idea came from the role model of our own left-wing solo general practitioner, who managed most of our family's medical needs. I would be my own boss, autonomous—free from political interference. I would be safe! This interpretation is one that has emerged over many years. At the time, I do not remember clearly articulating this analysis. Although I think it is true, at least at the psychological level, it may be one that I have assembled after the fact.

Physician independence? This view was more than a little naive. Whereas most doctors may have been independent entrepreneurs in the early to mid-twentieth century, the life of most physicians today is very much dependent on other forces, from insurance companies to governmental regulations. Today, a physician's independence is vastly curtailed.

I am certain, however, that my father's dependency on his bosses, both benevolent and malevolent, was a major factor in my choice to be "the boss" throughout my career, always as head of the Department of Family Medicine in numerous facilities. I now recognize a paradox, in that I really do not much like administration, yet I did it all the time, always as "the boss." Even in my medical training I followed this pattern, serving repeatedly as a chief resident. Although I enjoyed the administrative jobs enough to work at them seriously, I liked the role less than other activities that I might have undertaken. So why do I take on an administrative role if I dislike it so much? Because I would rather do something that I don't like very much than be subservient to somebody else. Thank you, Joseph McCarthy, US Army Intelligence (oxymoron), the FBI, et cetera.

7. OBERLIN COLLEGE AND PREPARING FOR MEDICAL SCHOOL

It was no accident that I chose Oberlin College. It was the first college to admit Black students, one of the first to admit women and a stop on the Underground Railroad, where escaping slaves from the South were hidden and protected. Oberlin fit nicely with our family values. Besides, it had an outstanding conservatory of music, and I planned to continue seriously playing my clarinet.

At Oberlin I found pre-med students competitive and narrow-minded, and for the most part I avoided them. I majored in political science and international relations, taking the bare minimum for entrance to medical school. While pre-med students were taking calculus, I could barely survive college algebra. In my political science classes, I occasionally used *I.F. Stone's Weekly* as a source for my papers. We read it regularly at home and had family discussions about the dissonance between Stone's reporting and what we read in conventional newspapers. I.F. Stone was a well-regarded left-wing writer, whose articles were well researched and a unique resource, a reality still appreciated today. My primary political science professor, an acknowledged very conservative refugee from Hungary and Soviet repression, gave me a lower grade for using this source.

As I had taken the bare minimum of the sciences and math needed to apply to medical school, it was not clear to me that I would ever be successful in gaining entrance. To hedge my bets, I was also preparing for law school. I could relate to books and films featuring the lawyer fighting single-handedly for justice against a heartless society. *To Kill a Mockingbird* was a good example. Law was another field where I imagined (falsely) that I would be independent, free from forces that could injure me.

But to get into medical school I had to suffer through physics and organic and physical chemistry, which were particularly rough. I managed, barely, because of the generosity of my brilliant roommate, the late David Sigman, for whom science courses were a breeze. In the end I took the aptitude exams for both law and medicine. I scored a few points higher in medicine than law, so I applied to medical school.

I had a generous swimming scholarship to Oberlin and thus had to spend endless hours in the pool, especially for the two years when I was captain of the swimming team. I had imagined that I would keep up my clarinet along with my swimming and studies. But because I was trying to keep up the clarinet while I was also obligated to swim, I was unable to compete with serious musicians in the Conservatory of Music, who practised their music many more hours than I could. Used to being first chair clarinet in high school, I soon found myself second and then third chair. This injured my self-image as a serious musician. And I was only a marginal "star" of the swim team. I did well in the group of mostly small Midwestern colleges, but we never could compete with the serious Ivy League powerhouses.

Frustrated by my comparative ineptitude in clarinet, I dropped clarinet and immersed myself in my studies, swimming and political activities, only picking up the clarinet forty years later, when my mother asked me to play for my parents' sixtieth wedding anniversary. Only this time I chose to play klezmer, rather than the classical music that I could no longer manage. Then the kids asked me to play at their weddings. Then I played my clarinet at my parents' memorials, until, lacking motivation, I again put it away. I am now trying to resume playing and even learning some new music, and for the first time in sixty years taking clarinet lessons.

Many years later, I learned that the CIA was actively recruiting at Oberlin, and apparently the FBI had strategically placed operatives in many classes. They were present at many political events—even folk-singing hootenannies in private homes. It was common knowledge that the CIA was recruiting at Harvard and Yale, but Oberlin? Left-wing Oberlin? Of course Oberlin. Who would suspect? As an aside, Jerry Rubin, one of the founders of the Yippies, lived a couple of doors from my dorm room. I remember him as a quiet kid who always wore a bow tie. Who knew?

As a political science major, one of the highlights of the program was Washington Semester. For an entire semester a selected six would go to Washington with our supervisor to study the workings of the US government. The program was tightly orchestrated, with time to spend in each of the houses of Congress, the Supreme Court and the study of the functioning of the presidency. Problem: one of the six of us was Rosemary Anderson, who, as it happened, was Black. It turned out that Washington in 1959 was a segregated city. We had planned to live together in a residence rented by the college. At the last minute we learned that Rosemary could not live with us. She would have to live in a Black residence. We six took a vote on what to do, easily deciding that we would abandon Washington Semester. Given recent events in the Trump presidency in 2017, looks like not much has changed.

Although I was pleased with my choice of Oberlin, I felt rather tentative socially. At a deep level, I felt unable to fully engage, particularly in political activities, because of a fear that began when I experienced the trauma of seeing my parents at extreme risk of exposure or jail for their politics. I expressed my political beliefs cautiously. Because of my dual life, there were some holes in my social development. Perhaps to fill this gap, at age twenty-one, in my senior year, I was taken with Irina Malbin, who was nineteen and in her second year. Irina was also the child of lefties. She was an attractive, gentle and sensitive young woman who was studying art as her major and was a fine painter—another link to my artistic family.

Our relationship soon became serious. I met and liked her parents and their circle of friends in Portland, Oregon. It really felt like home. I could speak my mind and discuss our shared interests, attitudes and beliefs. Irina's father was a radiologist, her mother a gifted pianist. My first sexual experience was with Irina. I think I had a rather puritanical idea that marriage was expected after sexual relations, so midway in my senior year we got married, moved out of our college residences and set up housekeeping. In those days, undergraduate marriage was virtually unknown. To supplement my Oberlin swimming scholarship and help with my parents' finances, I taught swimming and ran waterfronts in the summer, and worked as a head waiter in Oberlin dorms. In a fascinating turn of events, when we married, Irina and I were called into the office of Mary Dolliver, dean of women, who was in charge of dining halls. She was an imposing figure who always reminded me of the male actor Alastair Sim, who played house mothers and other female authority figures in many British films of the 1940s and '50s. Dean Dolliver was responsible for the rule that when men were visiting in women's dorm rooms, the door was to be open and each person was to have one foot on the floor. Dean Dolliver, tongue firmly in cheek, congratulated us on our marriage and fired me. "I know it feels harsh," she said, "but I am doing it for your own good," explaining that "married couples ought to eat together." The net effect was to create even greater financial strain on the marriage. Nevertheless, from my naive point of view, we were doing well as a couple. Irina continued to study art and paint.

At the fiftieth anniversary of my Oberlin class, I stayed at a student dorm with my brother, Henry, also an Oberlin graduate. The dorm was coed, as were all the dorms. There was a shared bathroom and shower. No particular attempts were made to separate the sexes. My, how things had changed.

8. MEDICAL SCHOOL

BECAUSE I HAD TAKEN ONLY the bare minimum of the science and math requirements for entry to medical school, I knew that getting into *any* medical school was going to be tough. I didn't really want to go there, but nevertheless I went for a medical school interview at Syracuse, just in case everyone else turned me down. I chose Syracuse specifically because I had an "in." My wife's father had gone to medical school with Julius Richmond, the dean of the Syracuse medical school, who later became Surgeon General of the United States.

It was a snowy Saturday morning in late 1959 when I presented myself for my medical school interview, having flown up to Syracuse on a two-engine plane on the now-defunct Mohawk Airlines. It was a bumpy ride. I spilled my coffee on my suit and arrived in a snowstorm with no boots for the slushy street or proper cold weather clothing. Freezing and wet, I trudged up to the medical school for my interview, only to find the door locked. I'd been shivering in the entranceway of Syracuse medical school for thirty minutes when a cheerful dean of admissions opened the door. After a pleasant interview, the dean told me that I was in. This was before the days of admissions committees operating with strict guidelines. But the dean was puzzled by my medical aptitude tests, explaining that I had scored in the ninety-fifth percentile for English and the twentieth percentile for math, results that he was sure could not be correct. With such scores in math he could not fathom how I got through chemistry and physics and the other pre-med sciences at Oberlin.

Would I mind, he said, redoing the tests? As it happened, he was one of the people who devised the national medical aptitude tests, and he was sure that there must be some kind of mistake. What could I say? He put me in a cubicle where I sat, cold and tired with wet shoes and pants, and I redid the test. Results: ninety-fifth percentile in English and twentieth percentile in math. Again, he expressed amazement that I had gotten through the pre-med sciences and said: "As I told you, you can come to Syracuse medical school, but I would not advise it, as you will almost certainly fail. I recommend that you apply to Case Western Reserve medical school." He made this recommendation after sensitively exploring my views on social medicine.

Case, in Cleveland, was already on my list of possibilities. The Syracuse dean explained that Case had a new curriculum that emphasized the social sciences as well as the biological. After a discussion of my values and hopes for future practice, he explained that as Case was trying to produce a socially committed physician, he felt that the school was more suited to my philosophy and approach to medicine.

Oberlin College did not allow cars, so I had a motorcycle, but for this import-ant interview I took the bus the sixty kilometres from Oberlin to Cleveland. The dean of medicine, Dr. John L. Caughey Jr., was a unique individual who had been personally shaping Case medical school as a new model. He was a reformer and developer of problem-based learning. Incredibly, he personally interviewed every applicant over decades. To introduce clinical medicine and social issues early, every new medical student was assigned a pregnant woman and was expected to attend her birth and continue to follow the family throughout the four years of medical school. I was intrigued by the prospect of following a family throughout pregnancy, birth and beyond. Based on the kind of physician Case was trying to produce, the school looked perfect for me.

The interview with Dr. Caughey was a relaxed and pleasant affair. I felt an instant bond with this reformer. "Mr. Klein, you can come here, and I would be pleased to have you, but in my opinion the preclinical years will be very difficult for you, and unfortunately you may wind up failing. In my opinion, you ought to apply to Stanford medical school. Stanford has developed a new five-year curriculum designed to produce an MD-PhD, physician-scientist. You, however, will need the five years just to get through. And as it happens, I am a Stanford alumnus, and I often do interviews for Stanford. With your permission, I will call my colleague, Dean Robert Alway, and see what I can do." And so he did. With me sitting across the desk from him, he called Dean Alway, told him my story and his opinion that Stanford was where I ought to go. He put down the phone and said: "You're in." So just like that, the long anxious wait to see if I was going to be a doctor was over. My relief was inexpressible.

In retrospect, this story seems unbelievable. Many years later, I found myself a member of the McGill University Faculty of Medicine Admissions Committee, where the committee made decisions collectively, as is the case in all medical schools today. However, during the time that I was a member of the committee, virtually all admissions to McGill were based on marks. Anytime I found an interesting student, especially one with a strong social conscience, often an older candidate, because of lower marks in the classic pre-med areas they didn't get in. I resigned soon after joining the committee, as I was looking for a different kind of future physician than was admitted to McGill at the time. It felt like my role on the committee was only to weed out the psychotics and convince the stars to come to McGill rather than Harvard. Everything else was decided by marks.

I am certain that if I applied to any medical school today, I would never gain admission and I would not be writing this story about my life as a doctor.

As predicted, I barely survived the first years of the basic medical sciences. Biochemistry and statistics were particularly difficult. As in my undergraduate studies at Oberlin, I got through because of the help I received from several of my generous, well-prepared classmates, some of whom already had their PhDs in the biological sciences. Physiology, pharmacology, cell structure and function, and anatomy were not too difficult. I recall anatomy as a social event. Four of us shared a single cadaver, a middle-aged woman whom we came to appreciate for all that she taught us, while the group dissection process brought the four of us together as a team of collaborators. Working together in this way we became close friends. Although I struggled with the sciences that required math, overall I loved medical school. I actually liked some of the very subjects that gave me the most trouble, as I could easily see why I needed to master the full curriculum to be an effective physician.

Softening the hard work of the first two years, I developed close friendships with some of my professors, particularly Dr. Robert Greenberg, a pediatrician-endocrinologist, who became a confidant and my first mentor.

Whereas most married medical students kept to themselves and had few contacts outside of their marriages, I had many good friends in my original and the following class, married and unmarried, and have happy memories of those days. Most of my classmates saw our marriage as exemplary, and one in particular claims to have married and had a child because we did. Another medical student and his wife who became close friends with us thought of us as role models, despite their own tumultuous marriage. Did they ever have it wrong. Socially immature, I was oblivious to the developing cracks in our own marriage.

Opportunities for recreation were everywhere near Stanford, and at times it was hard to concentrate on medical studies when the sun was almost always shining. I was a competent free diver and regularly dove for abalone on the coast. A favourite activity was to join with friends on an ocean adventure. We would walk through artichoke fields, pick a few, and then move on to the ocean, a preferred spot being the site of an abandoned coast guard station that had been taken over by California sea lions. We collected mussels and clams, and dove for crabs. The thousand-pound sea lions were not at all pleased with our presence. They were fond of looking at us directly in the face mask and occasionally bumping us or even biting. We would cook up our ocean bounty in white wine, garlic and seawater. My mouth waters just writing about it.

Although I was pleased enough to get through the basic sciences, it was clear to me that I was not a star. Therefore, I was surprised to be considered a potential summer student for Dr. Arthur Kornberg, who had received the Nobel Prize for synthesizing DNA. The planners for the newly redeveloped Stanford medical school recruited the best medical and basic scientists they could find, including Dr. Kornberg. These leaders would inspire and train physician-scientists, many of whom would become MD-PhDs, who would in turn become leaders across key fields in medicine and related sciences. Rather than passing on the laboratory work to their graduate students, the prizewinners themselves were expected to be readily available and inspire the medical students in the lecture hall and in small group lab work. As part of my experience, I got to synthesize DNA under the supervision of Dr. Kornberg himself.

It is important to say that, although Dr. Kornberg was a brilliant scientist, he was rather too brilliant for most of us and at times impatient with mere mortals. Fortunately, Dr. Kornberg's grad students were patient and managed to explain what we missed in the lectures. The medical students around me in the lab did understand biochemistry and openly shared their understanding with me, quite the opposite from the usual stereotype of competitive medical students.

Surprisingly, in June, at the end of our first year, Dr. Kornberg came into the lab and tried to entice us to spend the summer working with him. To do so would have been an outstanding opportunity. He began at one end of the lab with John Johnson. Modest and soft-spoken, John expressed his appreciation for the offer but explained that he was already committed to work with the chairman of the department of pediatrics, on the study of the diving reflex of California sea lions. John later succeeded Bob Greenberg as chair of pediatrics at the University of New Mexico.

Dr. Kornberg next approached Herb Kaiser, who held a PhD in pharmacology, who explained that his summer research was already committed.

Inexplicably, he next came to me. He must not have understood who I was or how unsuitable I would have been as a trainee. Nevertheless, with a straight face, I said how appreciative I was for the offer, explaining that I was already committed to teach swimming and run the waterfront at a bourgeois country club.

Next he reached Howard Fields, who explained that he was already committed to carry out his basic research on the giant crab neurotransmission process as part of his PhD in neuroscience. A similar process occurred with Peter (Jerome) Engel, who, like Howard, was working on his PhD in neuroscience.

This pattern of offering and being refused was repeated several more times until Dr. Kornberg reached the last person in the room: Loring Dales. Loring, a good friend, was known for his dry wit and killer one-liners. We all waited in anticipation of what Loring would say. "Dr. Kornberg," he replied, "this is the proudest moment of my life. I really wish I could come to work with you this summer, but I am already committed to run the kiddie train at Pacific Ocean Park." I don't know if Dr. Kornberg ever asked another student to work with him again.

Professor Joshua Lederberg received his Nobel Prize for fundamental genetic research, yet he lectured to us in basic genetics. He was a gentle man who enjoyed teaching. We students, of course, knew of his achievements, and some of my classmates had the privilege of working directly with him. Despite his desire to teach, his lectures, which contained mathematical concepts, were difficult for me, but thanks again to genetics grad students and my generous classmates, once more I squeaked by. However, over the summer and for months after, between the first and second years of medical school, we noted that Dr. Lederberg had disappeared.

When he suddenly resumed his lectures many months later, he looked like he had lost an enormous amount of weight, more than a hundred pounds. What was remarkable to us was that he had not bothered to have his clothing retailored. His pants were wrapped around one and a half times and were kept from falling down by a wide belt. His large suit jacket hung off him so that he looked like Charlie Chaplin.

To make matters worse, although his new weight was only about 160 pounds, he still walked like the more than 250-pound man that he was previously. As students sitting in the traditional steep lecture hall, it was hard to focus on his lectures while he paced up and down with his strange gait. This came to a head one day when, while pacing, he stepped into the trash can. Not only did he not stop to remove his foot from the trash can, he continued to clomp around while he went on lecturing, seemingly oblivious to the spectacle. How could anyone learn anything under those conditions?

9. THE STANFORD CLINICAL YEARS

I HAD SURVIVED THE PRECLINICAL years and now began to shine in clinical work with patients. As I was thinking about what field I would eventually choose, I was exposed to an excellent public health professor, who had had extensive medical experience in developing countries, and who encouraged students to experience medicine away from the ivory tower at Stanford. Perhaps it was a romantic notion of escaping from areas of medicine where I did not excel to ones where I would be more likely to be successful, but I began to think that I might go into public health or international health.

But what was most important to our future choices was to see our professors as human beings, physicians whom we could emulate. Each discipline had a different character. The surgeons, with exceptions, in many ways were like the arrogant stars of popular television programs like *Grey's Anatomy*. They were talented but narcissistic, impressive in their engagement in dramatic life-saving enterprises.

In my high school days I had initially thought I would become a surgeon; now I found myself attracted to other specialties with patient contact. Role models are everything, and for me it was pediatricians. I just liked the way they talked to children and parents. My preceptors were gentle and supportive, and gave us the supervised scope to become caring physicians. I was surprised they were that way, as Stanford Medicine was designed to produce the hard-nosed physician-scientist. Years later, at the fortieth and fiftieth reunions of my first medical school class, because so many had indeed become bench scientists with limited patient contact, some asked me what actual practice was like.

One of my first experiences in pediatrics is illustrative of the way we were taught to work with patients. For third-year medical students working in the pediatric outpatient department, the usual plan was for the medical students to take a history, do a physical examination and present the patient to the supervisor. My first patient of the afternoon was a ten-year-old girl whose complaint or concern was fainting. Actually, it was the parents' complaint. The story was a bit difficult to understand, so I invited the parents to sit in the waiting room so that I could talk with the girl alone. Crying, she explained that the family were Jehovah's Witnesses, that she was expected to go door to door on Sundays with her parents, distributing the publication *The Watchtower*. Her parents would ring the doorbell, and it was common for the householder who opened the door to be angry and often abusive, even swearing. This is when she would sweat and faint, and her father would catch her. After he laid her on the ground, she would slowly recover.

The parents verified the presentation. To me it seemed to be a classic vasovagal attack or emotional faint, in which the blood pressure suddenly drops. But unlike the usual response to a drop in blood pressure, which is to increase the heart rate to compensate, in a vasovagal attack there is no compensation. The blood pressure is low and the heart rate is very slow. The blood leaves the brain and the person faints. She would recover rapidly when in a horizontal position. It is a psychophysiological reaction, which can affect even tough guys exposed to blood, or so the stereotype goes. Whatever you do, don't try to get a fainter upright. The treatment is to lay the person down.

When I presented the case to my supervisor, he agreed with the psychophysiological reason for the problem. I suggested that we explain the mechanism to the parents and recommend that she stay home on Sundays. Normally, by age ten the children are expected to accompany their parents on these visits. Nevertheless, when a medical authority makes a strong recommendation, many "Witnesses" will follow it, even when it goes against their religion, as it removes from the parents the religious obligation in question. This kind of issue is much less important to the Witnesses than the well-known refusal to receive a blood transfusion.

At the follow-up visit, both the parents and the child were satisfied with the result. Although it was a simple case, this was my first experience with the importance of psychological issues that accompany many physical illnesses, and my supervisor, Dr. Luigi Luzzatti, was pleased with my approach.

10. CHIAPAS, MEXICO

IN 1963, HAVING SURVIVED THE preclinical years and beginning to taste the fun of clinical medicine, I decided to treat myself to a break from the structured life of a medical student. I contacted the Stanford Department of Anthropology after learning that they supported students as part of their research program. I received a grant to work in Mexico near Guatemala on a medico-anthropological project. It began as a summer student project, combining vacation with elective time for six months of continuous time. It was my first break from medical studies and a test for what I thought could be my eventual future role in international medicine.

The project was based on work that a researcher from the American Heart Association had done. He had studied hypertension among Bantu women in South Africa. His research showed that hypertension among Bantu women living under apartheid on reserves was rare, whereas among women in the major South African cities it was common; the Bantu diet was similar in both settings. Moreover, women planning to migrate to the city had intermediate levels of hypertension, between levels in the city and the reserves.

Women on the reserves were not the head of the family, whereas in the city they were. Thrust into an unaccustomed role, while their husbands mostly worked in the diamond and gold mines, the stress of being head of the household in the city was great. The theory held that stress was the causal factor creating the hypertension. The theory was to be tested in another setting, among Mayan communities in Mexico along the Pan-American Highway. It was hypothesized that Mayan communities deep in the interior would be hypertension free, whereas those undergoing cultural stress close to the highway would show the greatest hypertension, with hypertension rates following a continuum from high to low stress with distance from the highway. We expected to find blood pressure increasing with age, as was found in both developed and developing countries.

So off Irina and I went in a car jammed to the roof with medical equipment. We travelled down the West Coast through charming towns and some cities, like Mazatlán, which have since been forever altered by high-rises and the tourist trade.

We arrived at the US-Mexico border, never thinking I would have a problem bringing across the tools to measure blood pressure, examine basic urinary function and check the retina for evidence of severe hypertension. Although I had a microscope, a centrifuge and some other expensive equipment, what got me in trouble was a large box of more than one hundred conical cardboard disposable urine collection containers.

"You are going to do what with these containers?" asked the border agent.

In my best rudimentary Spanish, I explained: "People are going to urinate into the container. Then I am going to examine the urine under the microscope."

"Felix," the agent explained uproariously, "this guy says people are going to piss in these bottles."

Soon a group of five or six agents gathered around and made jokes about pissing into the containers. They removed me from the lineup and put me to one side, where we argued for an hour or so about the science associated with pissing in a bottle. I assumed they wanted a bribe, but pigheaded me, I was not going to provide it. In the early 1960s, as I learned later, containers of all types were rare and valuable in Mexico. In our age of disposable bottles, it may seem absurd, but the border agents may have just failed to believe me.

Finally, it dawned on me. I don't really need these damn containers. I am not doing a bacteriological study. All I need to do is use glass pop bottles and wash them out between subjects. I turned over all the containers to the incredulous border agents. In moments, we were on our way.

Passing through Mexico City and south on the Pan-American Highway, we finally entered Chiapas and the territory well explored by the Stanford anthropologists. Teopisca was a village in extreme transition. The population was about twenty thousand *mestizaje*, or people of mixed Mayan and Spanish descent. Although the physical features of the townspeople were strongly Mayan, they dressed in Western clothes and spoke Spanish, unlike most of the Mayans farther south in Chiapas.

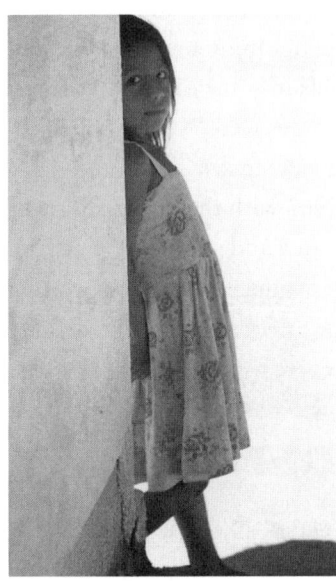

A young girl standing in a doorway in the Mexican village of Teopisca.

As my supervisor, John Hotchkiss, and I drove down the main street of Teopisca in the open yellow World War II vintage Jeep assigned to me, John stood up waving, while holding on to the windshield. We heard in Spanish, "Don Juanito, Don Juanito. He's back. He's back. Come here. Come here!" Door after door opened, the people greeting John ecstatically. I had the absurd notion that this was like the reception of the American troops liberating Paris, but John was truly loved in this village.

Dr. Hotchkiss was a Stanford anthropologist who had spent years studying drinking behaviour in this town and in the more southern Mayan towns near the Guatemalan border. He was known for his shared drinking with the "guys." Endeared to the town, and thoroughly integrated into life there, he had a local girlfriend, Lupe. He eventually married Lupe, and she moved with him to Stanford, where they had a lovely child, who, when John got to drinking a little too much would say: "Hey, *stupido*, cut it out." It worked.

Over a number of years, the anthropology department at Stanford had studied a variety of cross-cultural phenomena in Mayan transitional communities and had developed trusting relationships with key Mayan community leaders. John had also been so befriended by the Mayans of the region that he could open doors for us medical students for our various medico-anthropological projects and act as an advisor and troubleshooter. He identified and hired for us the *informante*, or translator-fixer.

Aquacatenango, the study town, was an hour away from the Pan-American Highway and an hour or so south of the nearest major town of San Cristóbal de las Casas. Aquacatenango was a pueblo of about one thousand people who spoke a Mayan dialect called Tzeltal. Adjacent communities spoke other related Mayan idioms, like Tzotzil, but although the ancient Mayans had written language, none had written languages in the 1960s.

Aquacatenango still remains one of the poorest and least-known villages of the area. Nearby villages on the highway like Chamula, Zinacantán and Tenejapa managed to work themselves into the booming tourist trade, and today there are even fairly well-developed hotels in some of those villages. At the time that I worked in the area, these villages were "sleepy" pueblos, little touched by outside or even inter-village influences. Today, it is hard for me to reconcile the area that we knew in 1963 with the Zapatista revolution of the 1990s, which involved the whole area and stopped the central Mexican government from exploiting the rich mining and other resources of the area.

The town was divided into two barrios, or neighbourhoods, roughly situated on either side of the adobe Catholic church, whose priest preached only in Latin and Spanish. Although the townspeople spoke Tzeltal, a few of the men spoke some basic marketplace Spanish. Generally, only the women attended church, and they comprehended nothing the priest said. Occasionally, a handful of men stood in the back of the church and understood a bit of

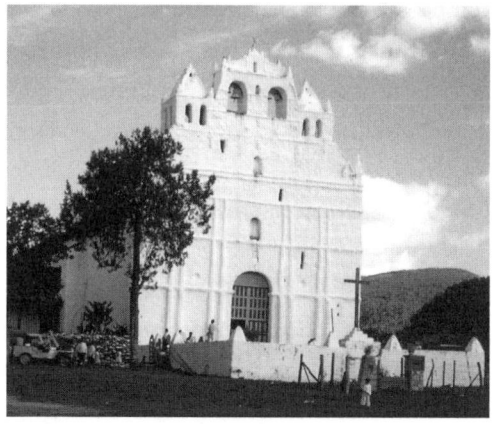

The church dividing the town of Aquacatenango, Mexico. The World War II–era Jeep that we were assigned for our student project is parked to its left.

what the priest said. But I was one of the priest's devoted followers. I used his preaching to help consolidate my Spanish. Aquacatenango was a very stressed town in transition, with the men usually leaving town to seek employment elsewhere. Reflecting the transition, townspeople dressed mostly in traditional clothes, but cheap Western clothing was beginning to appear. They practised both Catholicism and a local Mayan animistic religion.

The church was also under great religious stress. While the Catholic priests continued to preach in a language the locals did not speak, Mormons had been trying to entice Mayans over to their religion. The Mormons knew that to communicate and get converts, they needed to speak the Mayan languages. To accomplish this, they brought in trained linguist-anthropologists who lived with the Mayan people for extended periods of time so that they not only learned the local languages but created a written phonetic language. Then they created and distributed a phonetic Mayan Bible to people who for the first time had a written language. This powerful tool worried the Catholic priests throughout the region.

One day, standing in the back of the church, consolidating my Spanish, I learned that Mormons and Jews were the Antichrist, and that Jews were identifiable by the horns on their heads. Mormons were identified by the fact that they did not drink alcohol. I was not at risk, though I was Jewish, as I did not have horns and usually accepted a drink. But the Mormons were in some difficulty. The priest told the non-comprehending audience that if you offered an intruder a drink and he refused, then he was certainly a Mormon and should be driven out of town, or worse. Clearly, some of his message leaked out of the church.

So in my effort to prove my Catholicism, I began to regularly accept a drink. The anthropologists had published on the drinking behaviour of the Mayan communities and warned me of the dangers of too enthusiastically accepting social drinks. They prepared me by explaining that as the bottle of mescal (killer rotgut) was passed around, if you blew slightly into the bottle, bubbles would go up and give the illusion that you were drinking. Bob Armstrong, the other medical student on the project, felt that this was culturally dishonest. He dressed like a Mayan and was tipsy a good bit of the time. I felt that no matter what I did I would still be a gringo, so I just tried to be myself.

Irina and I lived with an extended Mayan family composed of a husband, wife, two young children and grandparents. We had our own room attached to the family compound. We slept on cots and had some minimal bedding and pots and pans. We ate with the family, a diet of tortillas and beans, which we supplemented with peanut butter and jelly and an occasional egg, piece of dried meat or fish. Cooking tortillas over a camp stove was not too bad. We

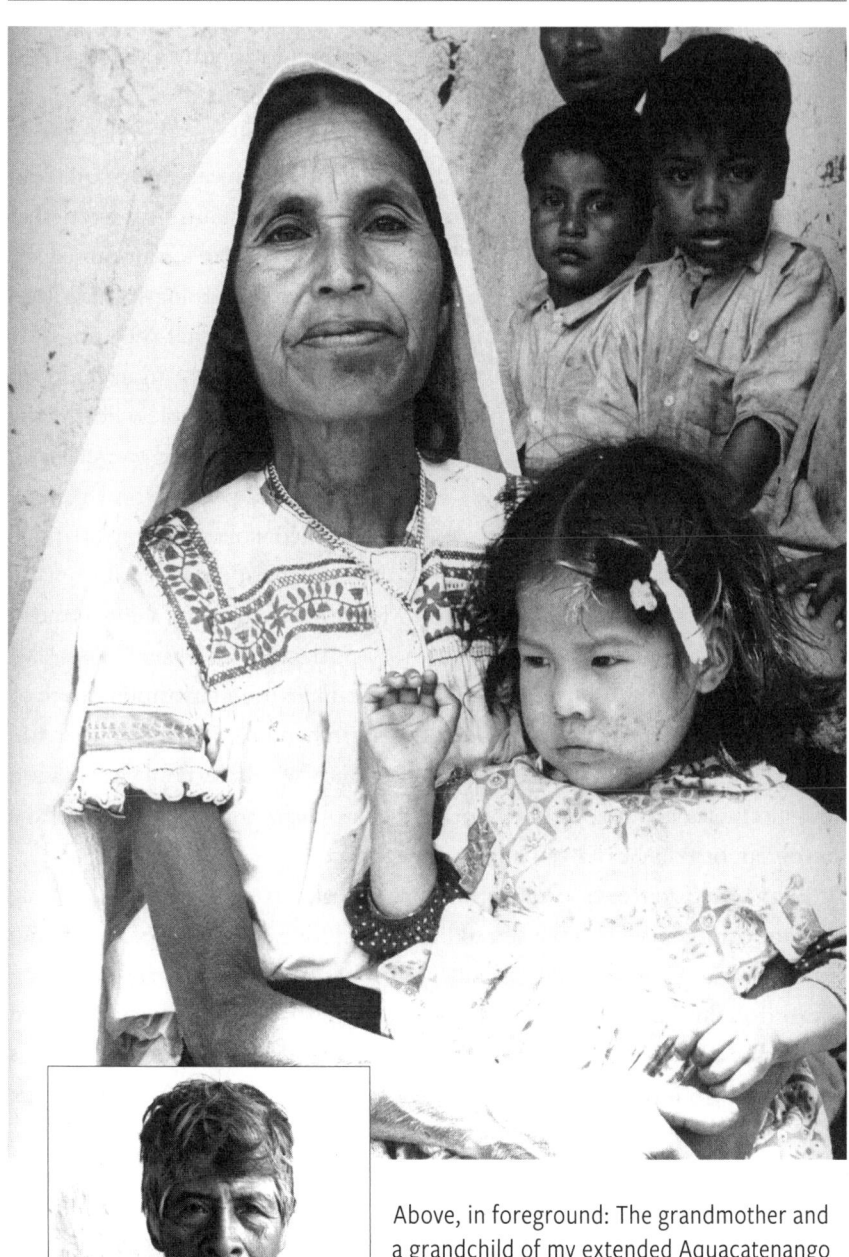

Above, in foreground: The grandmother and a grandchild of my extended Aquacatenango host family.

Left: The grandfather of the family with whom I lived in Aquacatenango.

occasionally went to San Cristóbal in our Jeep to eat a full meal and to go shopping. While I was immersed in my study, Irina was painting and experiencing life in this small community.

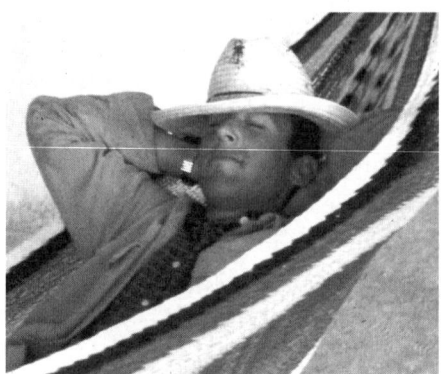

Me resting outside our house in Aquacatenango, which was located amid many cantinas.

One day during a San Cristóbal break, resting in the Stanford anthropologists' compound, we heard a frightening sound. Two yellow Mustang WWII fighter planes were diving, their engines screaming. We ran to the town square to see the fighters diving on a funeral procession that was being held in the central plaza. The dive-bombers were making low passes and scattering the mourners. What the hell was going on? We finally learned a complex story of love and intrigue. It turned out that a local man had been hitting on the wife of a member of the Mexican Air Force. He was murdered by the irate air force officer. The funeral was for the murdered man. It was not enough that he was murdered; he could not even be buried in peace.

Our Aquacatenango house was located in the centre of several *tocadiscos*, outdoor cantinas where music could be played for a peso per ranchera song. As a peso was a lot of money, usually the sponsorship of the song was shared among as many as ten men. The men would return late in the evening from their work and begin to unwind by sponsoring a 45 rpm single record, with all the contributing sponsors being named over the bullhorn loudspeakers mounted high on a pole. As there were only about ten to twelve family names in the pueblo, the sponsorship would begin with the announcement: "Good evening. This is Juan Aguillar Espinosa, drinking with my good friends Jose Aguillar Espinosa, Pedro Espinosa Espinosa, George Espinosa Aguillar…" after which the bullhorn would play the song while drunken workers added their singing and yodeling. Meanwhile, other cantinas were undergoing a similar process, seemingly aiming their speakers directly at us. Our house was located between three to four of these cantinas. The singing and sharing went on until two or three in the morning.

We tried to plug our ears, as did many of the townsfolk, as unhappy with the perpetual noise as we were, but complaining was out of the question. The danger to the potential complainant was the possibility of being named a witch if anything happened to the people making the racket. So the townspeople, especially the women, swallowed their annoyance and tried unsuccessfully to sleep. I would lie on my back and amuse myself by watching the rats running across the ceiling beams until finally I would fall into a fitful sleep.

The town had a small medical dispensary managed by a nurse, Vincente, who generously assisted me with my project. He was a pleasant colleague who shared his ideas and problems, and was a source of information on local folk remedies and practices. The federal agency responsible for the clinics supplied Vincente with antibiotics and anti-parasitic drugs. He had a microscope and a basic laboratory, and was on good terms with the populace.

Just prior to my arrival, the town had been visited by a major measles epidemic, an outbreak that had devastating consequences for the undernourished children of the town. There had been many fatalities and some children were left with hearing loss, chronic chest infections, chronic ear infections and the residual effects of the accompanying encephalitis, including a few children who were permanently brain-damaged. These measles complications are almost unknown in current Western societies, where measles and many other childhood diseases have been eradicated through modern immunizations.

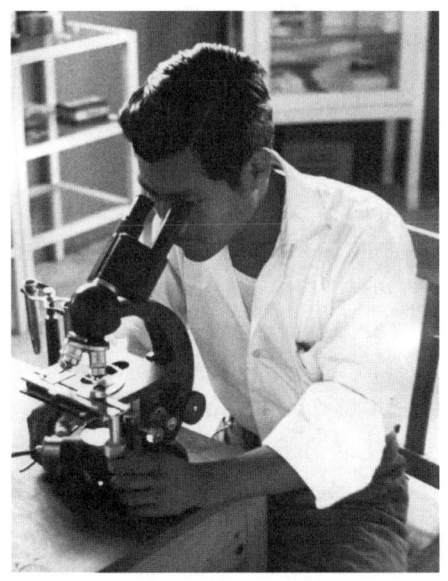

Vincente, the nurse who managed the small dispensary in Aquacatenango.

In the West, the very success of these immunizations has opened the door to vaccine deniers and allowed for a resurgence of previously eliminated illnesses.

My *informante* assisted me in finding community members so that I could study their blood pressure. My *informante* spoke Tzeltal to the subjects and marketplace Spanish to me, which I translated into written English for the project. To make a long story very short, I found absolutely no hypertension in any people in the town, young to very old. So our plan to measure the role of hypertension according to the stresses of being a transitional town was a complete failure. The very reason for the project for which I was in Mexico had disappeared. All that planning, all that medical equipment, all those urine containers—for nothing!

As I was wondering what I would do with the remainder of my time, the town experienced a major epidemic of typhoid fever. Many town members of all ages came down with typhoid. The likely source was a contaminated drinking water supply. There was one outhouse in the town, next to the church. Apparently, the priest used it. I must be repressing what we did for our own toileting needs, as it is bizarre that I cannot remember. Surely, we did not traipse across the road to the church every time we needed to pee. Vincente also got typhoid and was removed for treatment by the Indian Agency, but before Vincente left he gave me the keys to the clinic, where he had large supplies of chloramphenicol, an antibiotic that is effective against typhoid. Irina also got typhoid and, reluctantly, I had to treat her as well. Even then I knew that doctors ought not treat our own family members.

Here I was, a third-year medical student, the de facto medical officer of the town. I liberally dispensed chloramphenicol, and my patients did well, including Irina. Meanwhile, there were three *curanderos* also working against the epidemic, two young ones and one who I estimate was well over eighty years of age. *Curanderos* dealt with typhoid and other diseases by organizing a curing ceremony. Febrile diseases and most other diseases were thought to arise from "loss of soul." I'm oversimplifying, but loss of soul was thought to occur from "a fright" or at times witchcraft. An accusation of being a witch could lead to the accused being killed. It almost sounds like the Salem witch hunts in colonial Massachusetts. Curing ceremonies followed a defined pattern. They were organized to recover the lost soul.

The outcomes of the typhoid curing ceremonies by the town *curanderos* were not good. Several of the people of the town brought family members to me after failed curing ceremonies. My good results were not lost on the townspeople, as increasing numbers came to me for treatment. The two young *curanderos* never approached me, but the older *curandero* paid me a visit.

He explained that he knew that I was doing well with the medicines that I was dispensing and acknowledged that his results were not so good. He wanted me to supply him with the drugs I was using, which he said he would incorporate into his curing ceremonies. He told me that he often combined traditional curing with Western drugs. For example, he was regularly using the drug chloroquin as part of his curing ceremonies for malaria. He left with a big plastic bag of chloramphenecol. This was my first experience of working at the interface between Western and other types of treatments, sometimes called "alternative therapies."

Unfortunately, although Irina was cured from her typhoid, she developed a secondary severe yeast infection. I felt unwilling to continue to treat her on my own, so we took a trip to Tuxtla Gutiérrez, the major town in the region, so that she could see a gynecologist. The trip was hair-raising, as we negotiated the reverse route of our arrival to Chiapas, following the winding road down from the highlands to the planes, often with blind curves, around which Mexican drivers were inclined to cross the centre line. The Tuxtla doctor confirmed my diagnosis and Irina's treatment was successful, but it was a stressful time for us both.

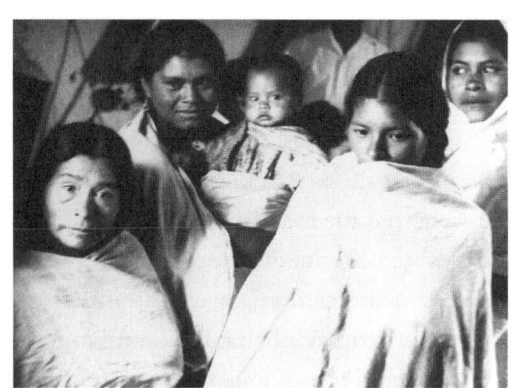

Women and their children coming to Aquacatenango's clinic for typhoid treatment.

A CURING CEREMONY

One afternoon, a man asked me to make a home visit to see his young child. The child was in a darkened room, curled up in the corner, wasted and unresponsive—clearly severely and permanently brain-damaged from measles encephalitis. I explained to the father that sadly there was nothing I could do. A week later, I was surprised but very pleased to be invited by the father to a curing ceremony. Although he had accepted that I could do nothing for the child, under pressure from his wife, he felt obligated to try one last thing. The ceremony was to be conducted by one of the younger *curanderos*, who I was told was a difficult and dangerous person. As I had hoped to see a curing ceremony before my time in Aquacatenango was over, with some misgivings, I accepted the invitation.

The curing ceremony began at about 11 p.m. under an almost-full moon. We walked around the town and the surrounding cornfields. About 4 a.m. we found the bleached skull of a cow. At this point the *curandero* announced that this was the place where, while working in the field with her mother, the child was frightened and lost her soul. We then walked quickly back to the family home. The comatose child was lying on a bed of straw. At one end was a Catholic cross and a lit candle. At the other end was a live chicken tied to a post. Palm fronds were arranged over the child in a tent-like structure.

We began to circle the child, singing in Tzeltal. After about fifteen minutes of circling, the *curandero* turned to me and asked for my watch, which he said was required for the completion of the ceremony. My heartbeat accelerated. I hoped that in the darkened hut my sweating went unnoticed. I knew the *curandero* was a manipulative hard case, so perhaps unwisely, I refused to give him the watch, saying that I did not think it was needed, as watches were not usually a part of curing ceremonies (nobody in the pueblo had one). At this point the *curandero* became enraged, kicked over the palm frond structure, inadvertently liberating the chicken, who jumped all over the hut, wings flapping. The *curandero* stated that the child would die and it was my fault. He pronounced that I would suffer for my action. He refused payment for the ceremony and left the house in a huff.

We were all stunned, and I was frankly terrified. Fortunately for me, given the area's history of violence to resolve disputes, the father quickly stated that this was very bad behaviour on the part of the *curandero*. Throwing his arm over my shoulder, he stated firmly that he knew that I was not responsible if the child died. He insisted that we all share a meal, which we did. The child died several days later. The *curandero* left town and did not return during my sojourn in Aquacatenango.

Several weeks later, a rather thin Vincente resumed his nursing duties at the clinic. It was time for me to return to Stanford to continue my medical studies. There was no question that the Mexico experience showed me that I could function as a doctor. The difficulties of the preclinical years were a distant memory.

11. ETHIOPIA: A TURNING POINT

TYPICALLY, MEDICAL STUDENTS' FUTURE PLANS are influenced by their most recent rotation through the specialties. Chiapas reinforced my plans to go into public health or international health. However, back at Stanford, clinical studies in internal medicine, pediatrics, psychiatry and surgery filled my time, but after the excitement and independence that I had in Mexico, returning to dry medical studies was a shock.

The third or fourth year is the time when most medical students are beginning to consider their future discipline within medicine—internal medicine, surgery, pediatrics, et cetera. Family medicine as an academic discipline had not yet been invented in the US, and I never saw a general practitioner (GP) in all of my training at Stanford. The field that attracted me most was pediatrics, not least because of my relationship with Dr. Bob Greenberg. Apart from appreciating his way with child patients and their parents, I was comfortable with his political views and how, despite them, he was able to somehow function in the usually conservative medical environment, though Stanford was more to the left than many medical schools.

Irina and I lived in a cockroach-infested former US Army barracks, hastily put up for the returning World War II veterans. Irina got a job at a local art school and I studied my brains out. When Irina became pregnant, we were delighted. We received care from a progressive obstetrician, who is still remembered today as a pioneer in what we now call family-centred maternity care. We just thought of him as a flexible, well-recommended doctor who seemed like a nice guy. When he suggested that Irina give birth on her side, rather than in stirrups—a radical thing in 1963—we went along with it. What did we know? In retrospect, this was my first exposure to another way of seeing birth. Episiotomy (a surgical cut designed to enlarge the vaginal opening to facilitate birth) was unlikely to be employed in that side-lying position. Irina gave birth to a healthy and much-loved girl whom we named Misha.

The positive Mexican experience had whetted my appetite for international medicine, and although my usual Stanford clinical studies were going well, I craved more international experiences. At the time, Stanford was a five-year medical school, whereas others were usually four years. In 1964, while I was in the early months of my fifth year at Stanford, I obtained an international scholarship award to study pediatrics at the Ethio-Swedish pediatric hospital in Addis Ababa, Ethiopia. This six-month stint involved three months of elective time and three months of holiday.

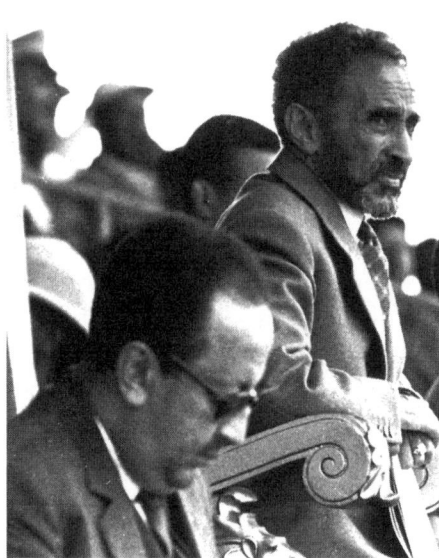

Emperor Haile Selassie at a soccer game, with the crown prince in the foreground.

This was when Haile Selassie was the emperor of Ethiopia, and life was a little tense because there had been several failed attempts to overthrow him. Just prior to our arrival in Ethiopia, in 1960, there had been a failed coup while the emperor was away visiting Brazil. His son, the crown prince, was involved; the rebels gave him the choice of cooperating or being executed. When the emperor returned, with his plane circling the airport, he broadcast that he was returning, that he was not afraid to die but was determined to remain their emperor in order to continue the work of "saving the country." This was the same emperor who during 1935–36 had stood up to the invading Italians and pled his case before the League of Nations. As his plane circled the airport, the emperor expected that the plotters would lay down their arms, which they did. The story goes that when Haile Selassie finally embraced his son, the crown prince, he said: "As your father I am pleased to see that you are alive and well, but I would be more proud to be attending your funeral."

These tensions made the foreign community jittery. One day a uniformed American soldier in a camouflaged Jeep visited me in the hospital compound. He announced that he was my "evacuation officer." He came from the American military air base, where one of our secretaries lived, married to a US soldier. At the time, all I knew of the base was that at Thanksgiving our secretary gave me a Butterball turkey. The base got all their food and water from the US.

The soldier explained that in the event of a coup, he would come for me in an armoured vehicle. I didn't even know that I had an evacuation officer. I explained that I was working for the Ethio-Swedish hospital and the Ethiopian government. Rather pompously, I explained that in the event of revolutionary activity, my duty would be to report to the hospital. Put out, he insisted that I exercise some minimal precautions, such as having containers of water and emergency food. As well, he cautioned me to fill my bathtub at the first sign of revolutionary action. At the time I thought, "What silliness."

Turns out I should not have been such a smartass. One evening, shortly after my evacuation officer's visit, I heard loud gunfire coming from the direction of the imperial palace. The palace was high above the hospital compound, in another part of town, screened from my view by a forest. I could see a red glow coming from the direction of the palace but could not actually see what was going on. Then, my anxiety increased because I saw an Ethiopian general who lived just outside the compound half-dressed and buckling on his sword. He was calling in the calibre of the heard weaponry by field telephone.

Anxiously, I called the phone company, asking of the operator: "Is there anything going on? I heard gunfire coming from the direction of the palace."

"Don't be foolish," was the reply. "Everything is normal."

I thought, *The rebels have taken over the phone company.* I started filling the bathtub.

Then I had an idea. I called a friend in the Peace Corps who lived above the palace. Laughing derisively, he said: "It's fireworks, you jerk, part of a celebration in honour of the visiting German prime minister."

Although I was only a medical student, my responsibilities in the hospital were great. I had colleagues to back me up most of the time, but I was in the extraordinary position of having an Ethiopian government-issued, full, unrestricted licence to practise medicine. Obviously, the country was desperate to get all the medical help it could. My position entailed undertaking normal duties and a regular rotation, just like the real doctors on staff.

The doctors were all pediatricians, one from Sweden, one from Holland and two from Ethiopia—one who had trained at the American University in Beirut and one not yet fully trained pediatrician named Demissie Habte. After completing his training in pediatrics at New York Hospital Cornell Medical Center, he became the first Ethiopian professor and head of pediatrics at Haile Selassie I University in Addis Ababa. While studying in New York, he and his wife, Seble, often spent time at my parents' home in New Jersey. I also had support from pediatric cardiologist, Professor Edgar Mannheimer, who had established the hospital. As I was the only student in the hospital, Dr. Mannheimer and the rest of the medical and nursing staff were determined that I would have a good experience and gave me lots of their time.

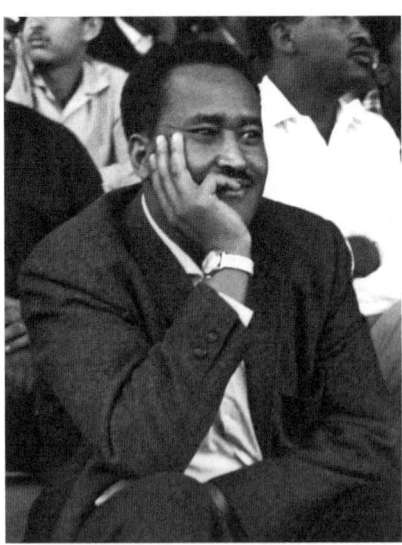

A key mentor in Ethiopia, Dr. Asrat Woldeyes, at a soccer game, where the emperor was also watching.

My duties included making regular ward rounds on the fifty in-patients, seeing up to sixty outpatients each morning (working with trained assistants, called dressers, who spoke one or more of the many languages). When it was my turn to be on call, one in four nights, I was in charge of the in-patient service alone overnight, just me and one nurse. My education in tropical and "Third World" medicine was of necessity rapid. I was taught, on the job, the diagnosis of the many diseases that filled the hospital and clinics. I learned to manage severe dehydration, meningitis, malnutrition, TB, diphtheria and shock. Doing so included a range of manual skills: lumbar punctures, suturing, intubation, respiratory therapies—skills well beyond the scope of a medical student at my level.

A wonderful man, Dr. Asrat Woldeyes, who was the only surgeon on staff of the general hospital attached to the pediatric hospital, requested that I assist him in surgery on a regular basis. Dr. Mannheimer agreed to free me up for that purpose. Dr. Woldeyes operated on virtually any surgical problem, from urological procedures to heart valve operations secondary to the effects of rheumatic fever, as well as a full range of abdominal procedures. As he was generally sleepless, he planned to teach me a few procedures so as to lighten his extraordinary load.

Thus I learned intubation and tracheotomy for the many children who arrived in extreme respiratory distress because of diphtheria and destructive laryngeal diseases. I did more than twenty of these operations, as well as simple procedures like appendectomies.

Tutored by the crusty, tough yet gentle Dr. Woldeyes, my learning curve was steep. In his caustic yet light-hearted way, he let me learn at my pace, despite my being slow. He allowed me to assist him, even when the operation would have gone faster if the nurses had assisted. Dr. Woldeyes helped me develop a sense of confidence that I didn't deserve.

There were no trained anaesthesiologists regularly on-site. There were anaesthesia nurses, but they did not manage small children. The chief and only anaesthesiologist in the hospital was a skilled Indian physician who was training nurse-anaesthetists for the entire country and was also establishing blood banking for all of Ethiopia. Consequently, he was almost never on the hospital grounds. So I had to do my own intubations of small children.

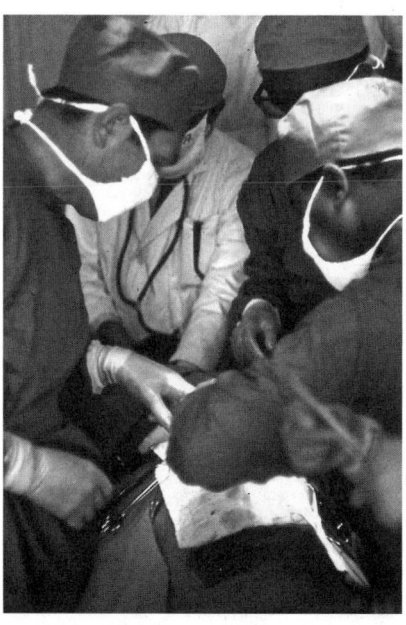

Dr. Asrat Woldeyes teaching me one of several procedures so that he could get some sleep. He was the only surgeon for Princess Tsehai Memorial Hospital, which was connected to the children's hospital.

I would normally have to intubate the child by passing a small rubber or plastic tube through the larynx. Then the nurse-anaesthetist would take over and ventilate the child while I would scrub out and scrub back in to complete the tracheotomy. With the airway tube in place, I could then safely do the tracheotomy over the tube. Finally, I would insert a metal tube and collar into the surgical opening in the trachea, through which the child could breathe.

The usual reason that I had to intubate a respiratory distressed child was for diphtheria or destructive airway diseases resulting from the cutting of the uvula at the back of the palate. This was done for "preventive" ritual purposes, as it was thought that a long or swollen uvula was the cause of many ills. Often this led to the virtual destruction of the larynx. In fact, there were times when the larynx was so destroyed that I had to do a rapid "slash-and-cut" tracheotomy without the benefit of passing an anaesthetic tube. This was a hair-raising procedure, as I had only a minute or so to do the tracheotomy, because the child would not be receiving oxygen until I finished the procedure.

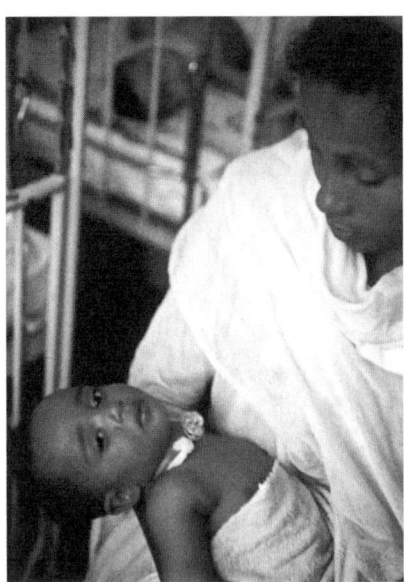

One of the Ethiopian children for whom I provided an emergency tracheotomy for diphtheria. His mother cared for him in the hospital, as did all the other mothers for their children.

One night, while I was alone on duty and deeply asleep in the on-call room, there was a loud banging on the door. Foggily, I opened the door to see a huge soldier in full uniform. Everyone recognized him as the security chief for the emperor. When he stepped to one side, behind him stood Emperor Haile Selassie himself, in whose arms was a ten-year-old boy, the son of the crown prince. The child was unconscious, pale and blue and having great difficulty breathing. I rushed him to the operating room, while somebody else called for the anaesthesiologist, who I was sure would be away, as usual.

The child clearly had epiglottitis, a severe swelling of the epiglottis at the entrance of the trachea, which was blocking his airway. The swelling was so great that I doubted I would be able to pass a breathing tube through the inflammation. But that night the gods were with me. This time, the anaesthesia chief was sleeping on the compound. With some difficulty, he was able to intubate by passing a very small two-millimetre tube, which secured an airway and moderated the emergency. His intubation allowed me to do a slow, careful cosmetic tracheotomy that would leave hardly a scar. Standing behind me on a stool and looking over my shoulder was a very short emperor. It all happened so fast that I hardly had time to think about the drama and my role. I just functioned automatically.

In 2018 in Western countries, epiglottitis is disappearing, as the bacterial organism that causes it, H. influenzae, is protected against by routine childhood immunization. This organism also causes one of the most common ear infections and a severe form of meningitis, both of which are vanishing because of the same routine immunization. Today's vaccine deniers have no idea of this history and how they are exposing society to diseases that were long ago eliminated. To make matters worse, they continue to promulgate the false information, long ago discredited, that vaccines cause autism.

The ten-year-old upon whom I operated was Zera Yacob Amha Selassie, grandson of Haile Selassie. He later attended Eton College and graduated from Exeter College, Oxford. He lives in Addis Ababa and is regarded as head of the imperial family of Ethiopia. In the unlikely event that the monarchy is restored, he will become the emperor. I wonder what would have happened if our anaesthesiologist had not been available that night. The emergency operation on the grandson of Emperor Haile Selassie was dramatic enough, more so because I was only a medical student pushing the limit of my skill set. I never thought to share my status as a medical student with the emperor.

The emperor was notorious for watching Dr. Woldeyes operate on his many relatives. The story was that he once said that if he were not the emperor, he would have liked to have become a doctor. Having met the grateful emperor on the occasion of the emergency tracheotomy of his grandson, we were "old friends." The emperor often brought sick children to the hospital. Typically, he would be driving around the countryside in one of his several Rolls-Royces, and he would find a desperately sick child, which he would bring to us. This created some problems, as inevitably that child would be so ill that they would need a private room. We had no private rooms, so other children would have to double, triple or quadruple up in other rooms. After all, this was the emperor's patient. Often, the child was so sick that survival was remote. He even found a child who, it turned out, was suffering with insulin-dependent diabetes. A lovely girl, she was relegated to living perpetually in the hospital, as insulin therapy was out of the question in her small village.

After I returned to Stanford to continue my training, a series of coups occurred in Ethiopia. Dr. Woldeyes refused to cooperate with the thugs who were then running the country and who ultimately jailed and killed the emperor and many members of his family. Earlier, he had formed a new party opposing the People's Revolutionary Party that ran the country. Dr. Woldeyes was put in jail, where he developed serious heart disease. The rulers of the country refused to let him out of jail to receive the needed treatment abroad. He was finally released from jail to get the necessary operation after Amnesty International intervened. He died in a Philadelphia hospital at age seventy-one after complications from heart surgery, probably because of delays in his treatment. Throughout all the political chaos, he remained Haile Selassie's personal physician and, before being deposed, was dean of Haile Selassie I University medical school. As an army surgeon he was known for insisting on caring for soldiers on both sides of the war between the north and south of Ethiopia, a position that the leaders of Ethiopia condemned. His principled and determined life reflects the man and teacher I knew and loved.

12. MIDWIFERY INFLUENCES

ALTHOUGH I DID NOT KNOW it at the time, midwives would play a major role in my future life as a doctor and researcher. When I was taking my turn on duty in the Ethio-Swedish pediatric hospital, and after the children were put to bed, it sometimes got very quiet. As the pediatric hospital was connected to the general hospital through a short tunnel, and because as a keen student I took every opportunity to learn, I would sometimes go through the tunnel to enter the maternity suite, where midwives would supervise me "catching" babies. Because I had not yet taken the conventional obstetrics and gynecology student rotation at Stanford, what the midwives taught me I saw as normal. Supporting women without technological interference, without using routine episiotomy and employing the techniques for natural pain relief just seemed the things to do.

Since I was thoroughly immersed in the life of the hospital and learning at a rapid rate, it became clear to me that six months was not enough time. My education in Addis Ababa was profound. I was involved in clinical care and research, and fully engaged in the work of the hospital, and, rightly or wrongly, I saw myself as needed. I petitioned the Stanford dean to allow me to stay another year to make a full year and a half in Ethiopia. This was granted.

As you can imagine, my life in the pediatric hospital was exciting—a medical student independently doing things that normally would be done by a much more senior physician, and certainly much later in training. One of my occasional duties was to fly on an old World War II vintage DC-3 to one of the outlying centres in another province, where I would do sick call and bring back patients to Addis Ababa who needed more than I could offer. Then I would return to do sick call a week or so later, ideally bringing back with me the people whom I had previously evacuated.

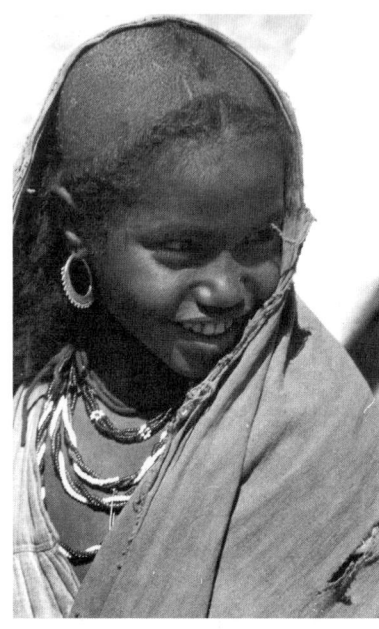

A young Tigre girl I saw in the clinic during one of my visits to a remote settlement in Ethiopia.

One memorable experience involved participating in the maiden voyage of a flat-bottomed aluminum boat to be used by the health officer in Gambela, in the south of Ethiopia near the border with Sudan. When the Baro River, which flowed south toward Sudan, flooded, roads were impassable, so for many months of the year the Gambela health officer could not reach the downriver small health units under his responsibility. The *African Queen* was loaded into the DC-3, the bench seats having been removed or turned up. The boat was then turned on its side while the cargo of chickens, goats, and crates and the rest of us were piled up around it.

The plan was to deliver the boat to Gambela, teach the health officer to operate the two outboard motors, and then travel downriver to the isolated health units, bringing supplies to support the minimally skilled dressers at these units. This we did, little realizing that there was a full-scale war in progress between the largely Christian nomadic Nubian tribesmen, who lived mostly in Ethiopia but crossed the border when they followed their cattle, and the central Muslim government of Sudan. On the way we had encountered rebels armed with World War I rifles. To save fuel for the return trip, we mostly drifted downriver, employing the motors only to avoid snags or deal with the current.

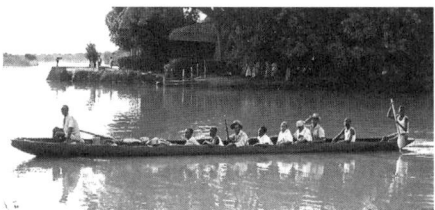 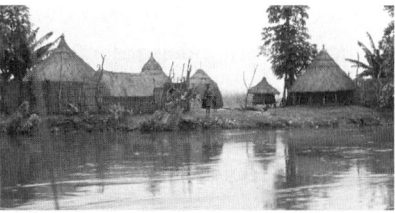

Flooding that occurred for several months each year made it impossible for a Gambela health officer to reach his health stations.

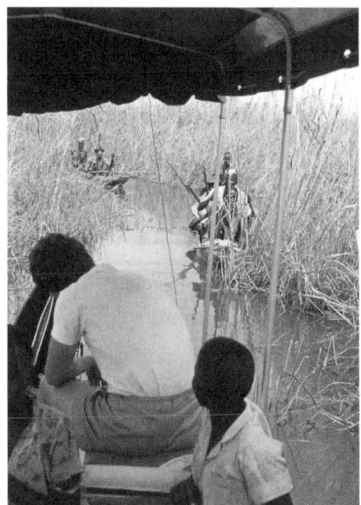

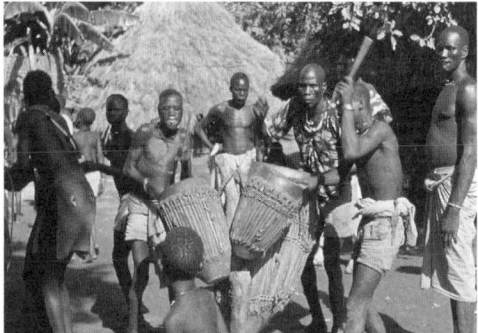

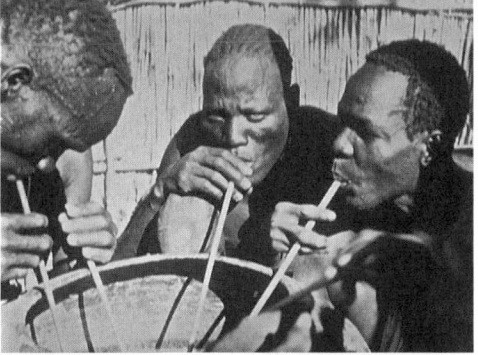

Above: Armed tribesmen in dugout canoes. This photo was taken from aboard the *African Queen*, the aluminum boat with a canopy designed for the Gambela health officer.

Top right: Villagers in the middle of a celebration, encountered on my river trip in southern Ethiopia.

Middle right: Celebrants drinking during festivities in Gambela.

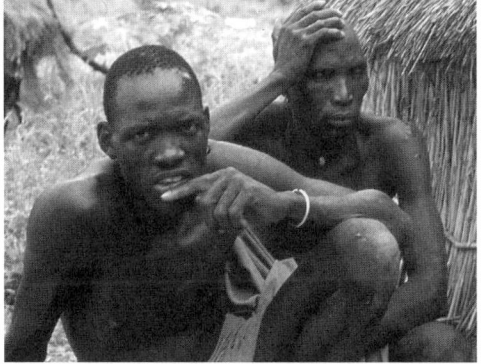

One day, with the river in full flood, making it impossible to know exactly where the border was located, a small gunboat fired upon us. It was noon. We had inadvertently blundered into Sudan in the middle of prayers. After things settled down and we explained our business, we were welcomed into the border stockade. The military officer in charge of the border post had been educated at the American University in Beirut and spoke excellent English. He invited us for tea.

We were a strange group: a non-religious Jew, a Christian missionary doctor-surgeon and the Gambela health officer. The officer in charge harangued us with war stories and told us that the tribesmen were supported and armed by the Israelis. I kept my Jewish identity to myself, but I thought that the story was far-fetched and just part of the usual pattern of blaming the Jews and/or Israelis for everything. On return to Addis, I learned that it was true. In retrospect, our naïveté was monumental. We were fortunate to have survived the episode.

On another occasion, I was assisting a missionary surgeon in another province, when he kneeled by the operating table to pray before the operation. Through an interpreter he said that if the operation was successful, he expected the patient to convert and join his Christian church. If the operation failed, it was God's will.

The hospital in Ethiopia was a wonderful setting to learn about diseases that affect children, specifically diseases that were endemic to the area. Protein-calorie malnutrition (kwashiorkor) presented regularly at the hospital. Treatment was feeding an appropriate nutritional mix. Some children were so sick that we could not save them. All diseases were of great interest to a medical student, but I developed a particular interest in rickets, because of vitamin D deficiency. Rickets was a major problem in Ethiopia. But why? Sunshine was abundant, so vitamin D should have been synthesized with ease in the skin of the children. Ethiopia used to boast being a country with "thirteen months of sunshine." Anthropological theory was that dark skin blocked the sun and protected against too much vitamin D. But being dark-skinned also could, under certain conditions, put you at particular risk of acquiring rickets.

We know that the first peoples were Black and became established at the equator. As people migrated toward northern climes, survival was possible only if one was lighter skinned, as synthesis of vitamin D in the skin was adequate only for fair-skinned people, like those from Scandinavia, who did not get rickets even if they received very little sunshine. The dark-skinned Inuit of the North are the exception that proved the rule. They did not get rickets because, rather than synthesizing vitamin D in the skin, they ate their vitamin D from seal and fish oils. That was until European colonizers (Americans) hired Inuit as rangers to protect their interests from Russian intervention. The usual hunting and fishing sources of vitamin D were supplemented by purchasing food from the Hudson's Bay store. Then rickets arrived in the North, and vitamin D fortification of milk and foods was needed to prevent the condition.

But rickets in Ethiopia? It made no sense. Well before my arrival it had been determined that the cause was the practice of keeping children indoors to shield them from the evil eye. By the age of one year, the infant was thought to no longer be susceptible. Unfortunately, by that time, especially very dark-skinned infants already had the disease. Many lighter-skinned babies were able to synthesize enough vitamin D to avoid rickets, even if they had little sun. And rickets was much more than bowed legs. Rickets was life-threatening. The chest deformities contributed to heart failure, and together with generalized malnutrition and anemia, rickets was a catastrophe.

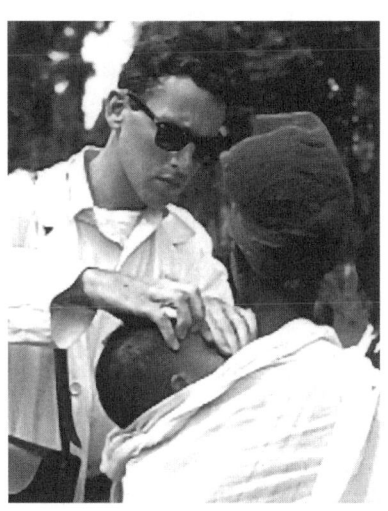

Me examining a child for rickets at a public health clinic in Ethiopia.

The Ethio-Swedish pediatric hospital organized many public health programs to educate people on the avoidance of rickets, but it was a hard sell, even with the carrot of free powdered milk distributed at public health clinics. In studying the disease, I benefitted from consultation with experts from the adjacent biochemical laboratory, the Ethio-Swedish nutrition institute.

In fact, the *Ethiopian Medical Journal* published my first-ever scientific paper, a study of a single Ethiopian family with two brothers who had severe vitamin D–resistant rickets. These two boys each had multiple fractures of long bones, as well as a collapsed chest and heart failure. I read up on the literature and treated them with a phosphate soup that I concocted based on my research, plus massive doses of vitamin D.

Although my paper on vitamin D–resistant rickets has held up over the years, my study and paper on the aminoaciduria of vitamin D–deficient rickets was unsound. After more than fifty years, I can say that the paper was of doubtful value and had many scientific errors. Nevertheless, these two studies launched my research career and anointed me with a passion to study the conditions that I encountered in my everyday practice.

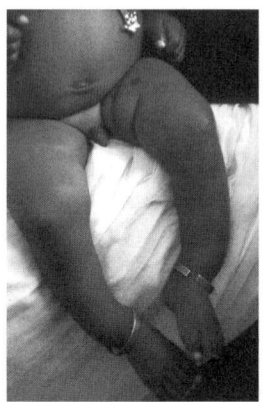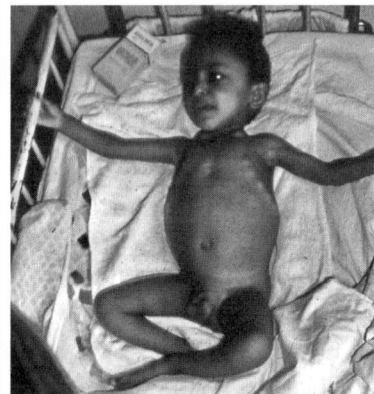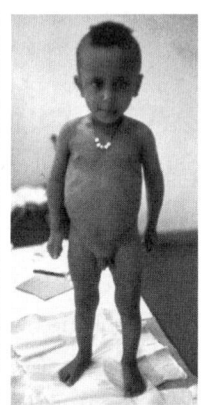

Left: This photo demonstrates a classic case of rickets in a child kept from the sun for almost one year. Note the bowing of the legs. *Middle:* A severe case of rickets including multiple broken bones before treatment with massive doses of vitamin D and a homemade phosphate mixture. The boy's chest shows the rachitic rosary sign—the joining of the cartilage and bone of the ribs is swollen in a bead-like pattern that resembles a rosary. *Right:* The same child six months later, after treatment for rickets.

TETANUS NEONATORUM: A TALE OF UNREALITY AND ARROGANCE

Although I did well in the care and treatment of many diseases, I could get carried away. Newborn tetanus was a common disease in Ethiopia. While I was working in the outpatient department, a child with newborn tetanus would present at regular intervals, usually at about a week of age. The newborn would normally have been born at home under the care of a village midwife. The umbilical cord would have been tied with horsehair, the source of the tetanus organism. Typically, the child would arrive too late for treatment to be effective. He would be stiff and usually having seizures. The child would die of respiratory failure. All we could do was refer the family to the health education department of the hospital in the hope that the parents would learn the cause of the disease and avoid it in the next birth.

Despite the almost certain death of these unfortunate newborns, being an overly keen and arrogant young student, I got it into my head that we ought to be able to save some of them. Studying the various approaches that were used, I located a protocol from a university hospital in Texas. Their cure rate was about 50 per cent. Therefore, in addition to sending parents to health education, I began admitting a few newborns with tetanus, despite the skepticism of the nurses. We managed their rigidity by paralyzing them with curare, treated their seizures and put them on continuous ventilation, the idea being to buy time until the antibiotics killed off the tetanus bacteria. Problem: No ventilators. Solution? Train the mother to ventilate her baby by hand, by squeezing a bag containing an oxygen mixture, until antibiotics and time could deal with the infection. The mothers learned how to do the ventilation, and the other mothers on the ward helped out when the newborn's mother fatigued.

Problem: There was only one nurse on duty overnight. She had the entire hospital to cover. She could only check on the tetanus patients and their mothers from time to time. The babies all died despite my brilliant impractical approach. The nurses, polite as ever, implored me to stop admitting these resource-exhausting patients. Their analysis was correct. We could save many more babies with other illnesses, while this doomed activity was using beds and taking staff away from patients who could be saved. I felt foolish, as well I should have. I stopped trying to postpone the inevitable.

THE ITALIAN TRADER'S CHILD

This time you might say that arrogance paid off. Late one evening, I was alone on duty when a child arrived near death. A week earlier he had been born at the Russian hospital in Addis Ababa, one of several hospitals run there by various foreign countries (Bulgaria, France, Britain, and others), all established in part to gain favour with the Ethiopian citizenry. The birth had been finally completed after prolonged vacuum extraction with a metal cup on the fetal scalp.

The child was comatose, deeply jaundiced and had a large boggy mass on his head where the vacuum had been applied. The skin was broken in the centre of the mass. It was at first unclear if the mass contained blood alone or pus as well from infection, the broken skin providing an entry point for bacteria. X-ray showed a skull fracture beneath the mass. Needle aspiration of the mass showed a mixture of blood and pus. Lumbar puncture revealed meningitis, undoubtedly the result of bacterial entry into the brain and then spinal cord. Blood cultures showed septicemia. I learned that the child was a much-hoped-for infant of older parents, traders from Djibouti, seven hundred kilometres away by single narrow-gauge railway. The couple had been trying to have a child for many years. The mother had come to Addis Ababa for the birth, and the father stayed in Djibouti.

I treated the baby's infection with broad-spectrum antibiotics, but the jaundice was so profound that an exchange transfusion was needed as well, but we had no equipment for the procedure. In modern practice, disposable plastic exchange transfusion kits are available in every well-stocked pediatric facility. In this case, I found myself putting together a homemade spaghetti-like exchange transfusion apparatus, made up of various tubes and valves stolen from other equipment. Blood donation was arranged from the mothers on the wards, and the procedure worked. The child slowly began to recover, though intact survival was unlikely.

Surprisingly, the child was really doing well, but on rounds a few days later I found he had become suddenly and unexpectedly worse. Examination revealed a loud, harsh to-and-fro heart murmur, classic for a ductus arteriosus. This results from the opening of a remnant of fetal circulation that almost always closes at birth and stays closed. In this case, for reasons unknown, it had reopened and the child was in serious heart failure. High concentration of oxygen, digitalis and mercury diuretics were the standard treatment at the time. I had just begun the treatment when the father finally arrived to meet his first-born son.

His response: "Stop everything. I do not want a damaged child." I was astonished by this response, especially given how long they had been waiting for a child, which was likely to be their only one. With the arrogance of a young doctor, not really a doctor yet, I pleaded for the chance to continue treatment and convinced the father to permit me to press on for a few hours, agreeing to stop if the treatment was not quickly effective. To my amazement, and in a testament to the resilience of little people, the murmur disappeared in a couple of hours. The child's colour rapidly improved. The treatment had worked and the ductus arteriosus had again closed. Within several weeks, the child was well enough to be on the train home to Djibouti. For several years, the parents managed to track me down at Stanford and later New York, where I would receive an annual bottle of expensive brandy. The accompanying card told the story of proud parents caring for a healthy child.

This case was one of the many in Ethiopia, and later in my career, when patients whose future looked bleak turned out healthy. These experiences shaped my future approach to both children and adults whose prognoses were poor. The resilience of the human organism, especially children, is remarkable, and the brain is so plastic as to be able to re-engineer itself after profound insult. This realization has led me to express a large degree of modesty in making predictions about the outcome of a variety of conditions.

What was the effect of the Ethiopian and Mexican experiences on my self-image and self-confidence? The powerful medical and research experience in Ethiopia was life-changing. My rapidly developing clinical and diagnostic skills, coupled with the acquisition of significant surgical and obstetric techniques, placed me in a position that few trainees at my level could hope to achieve. I was pretty full of myself. "Stamping out disease" was certainly satisfying, almost a high. It was also easy to develop an inflated notion of one's skills and importance, a heady, even addictive, mix. It was well known that this phenomenon could even affect experienced physicians, who after some years in this kind of environment had difficulty returning to their country of origin. To mitigate the problem, Swedish physicians were required to rotate home every three or four years.

One saving feature of the later portion of my stay in Ethiopia was my realization that many, even most, of the diseases that I treated were preventable through basic public health programs. Although I obtained great satisfaction from the curative work, I came to appreciate that the number of children with the diseases that I treated was infinite. My work, though important for the individual child under my care, was a drop in the ocean among the millions of needy children. The experience with rickets and newborn tetanus illustrated how health education would do much more good than me treating one child at a time—much as I enjoyed the role of saviour.

NEGLECTING MY OWN LIFE

Although I was saving lives and learning rapidly, my personal life was not going so well. Irina worked at the national art school, where she was profoundly unhappy. At home she felt isolated in the walled hospital compound where no one had small children.

Our toddler, Misha, had wonderful care from a lovely and gentle woman who came to our house every day. She would cook traditional Ethiopian meals with injera, a spongy, flat bread made from teff flour; clean the house; and talk to Misha in Amharic. Misha learned to walk in our little house. Her first word, apart from mama and dada, was the Amharic word for dog: *woosha*.

Absurdly, we also had our own personal guard, who had a guard dog—hence Misha's first word. We were treated with a level of support that was way out of proportion to our age and stage. It was hard not to have an inflated view of our importance. We tried to treat "our staff" with dignity, knowing we could never have afforded to pay for the same kind of help in North America. The money we paid the housekeeper and the guard supported layers of other workers, who in turn were paying their support people to look after their kids and homes, and so on down the economic line.

Although I was deeply satisfied with my medical work, I was unable to avoid the looming disintegration of our marriage. We were both immature and lacked the insight and tools to deal with our failing marriage, and we did not know where to turn for help. I buried myself in my work, and Irina buried herself in her art. Late in our stay in Ethiopia, Irina and I agreed to separate, making the remaining months very difficult. Although the Ethiopian experience was incredibly rewarding and life-changing in the very best way for me, the same was not true for Irina. I wish that Irina could have had a similarly positive experience. Our return to the US from Ethiopia via Europe to pick up our pre-purchased car was a kind of anti-honeymoon.

13. BRINGING IT HOME

After a year and a half in Ethiopia, it was time to return to Stanford to complete medical school, this time alone, Irina and Misha having returned to the family home in Portland. Thereafter began a regular pattern of visitation with Misha. Misha spent part of the summer and winter holiday vacations in New Jersey with me at my parents' home and later at all my future locations. Misha loved my parents and we all looked forward to those visits. Despite the four thousand kilometres between Portland and New Jersey, I was able to maintain a cordial relationship with Irina so that Misha could benefit from both families who loved her.

All I had to do to graduate from Stanford was a six-week clerkship in obstetrics and gynecology, some internal medicine outpatient clinics and a surgical subspecialty rotation in urology, plus some elective time. I began with the elective time, in which I cared for babies in the premature intensive care unit at Stanford University hospital.

The chief of the unit, Dr. Philip Sunshine, gave me serious clinical responsibilities, and we carried out an unpublished study on the establishment of diurnal variation in corticosteroid metabolism in premature infants. This required me to sleep in the nursery and take blood samples at regular intervals. I had to do my own analyses of the blood samples to measure the levels of corticosteroids produced by the premature infants' adrenal gland. I accomplished the analyses under the supervision of Dr. Bob Greenberg, my role model as a pediatrician and scientist. Initially, I so wanted to be like him, a bench researcher, that I was willing to work in a dark room in the basement while I did the analyses. But I learned that I hated the laboratory, which was so central to his work. We kept up our relationship even though, in the end, I followed a different path. Bonnie and I feel fortunate to have spent time with Bob and his wife, Maggie, a few months before Bob died suddenly while watching a live college basketball game. I marvelled at his positivity and determination, even though he was on supplemental oxygen in the years and hours before his death. Into his nineties, Bob still had many plans for the future and continued to try to make the world a better place for children and families.

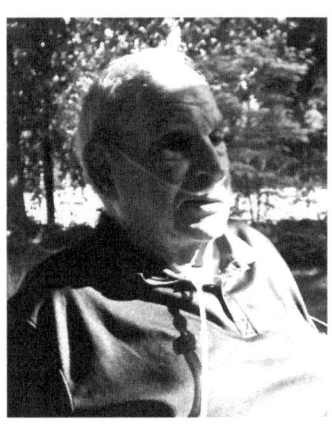

Dr. Bob Greenberg, my first mentor, in his late eighties.

Soon after my return to Stanford, I was paged to come to the pediatric outpatient clinic, where I met a woman who looked vaguely familiar. She was accompanied by a boy about three years old. She refreshed my memory of the case in which, as an early third-year medical student, I had played a minor, mostly observer role. Her ten-month-old boy had presented to Stanford with a huge liver and severe jaundice and pallor. I had done the initial assessment of the situation and presented my findings to my supervisor. On open biopsy it was clear that he had an aggressive, untreatable end-stage liver cancer, which also caused his severe anemia. His condition was destroying his red blood cells. My teachers determined that there was nothing to do. The abdomen was closed and the boy was sent back to his home in a rural setting with the admonition to love him the limited time he had left. Although medically I had nothing to offer, I had spent significant time supporting a distraught mother.

Here was that same boy, looking perfectly healthy. The mother had remembered me as a medical student and paged me to show me her apparently healthy son.

I was astonished. My jaw dropped, and I said: "What happened? How did you manage to get him well?"

She replied, "I found Jesus, and I divorced my abusive husband."

"Good for you," I replied. As young medical students we were more open and relatively unbiased. That is not always true. Some medical students, in their total identification with the "real medicine" they struggled so hard to learn, dismiss "soft" concepts, preferring "hard" science. A case like this can also shake the confidence of the learner and even cause him to question the very discipline he's chosen. Many early learners prefer to dismiss the "unusual case" as a fabrication or aberration. At the time, I cannot recall being more inquisitive or introspective about this miracle case. I just accepted it.

At the mother's insistence, a couple of fine needle liver biopsies were done. No evidence of tumour. Throughout my career in pediatrics, neonatology and, ultimately, family practice, I continued to be exposed to inexplicable cures, teaching me to be very careful about giving negative prognoses, even in the face of almost certain death or extreme disability. Giving an absolutely negative prognosis, I was to learn again and again, would demotivate the families of both small children and adults. Moreover, the plasticity of the human brain and the resilience of humans regularly proved the experts wrong, even when it was impossible to understand why patients got better when they ought not to, whereas others who ought to do well did not. What I was learning was that negative prognostication was something that families and loved ones never forgot, but a positive or even a wait-and-see-attitude, motivated the families and encouraged them to try to improve a dismal situation, which enhanced recovery. I wondered what this negativism was all about. Were we afraid to be wrong, to give false hope?

In my later practice, I often wondered why many of us tended to emphasize the negative, rather than the amazing capacity, from very small newborns to adults, to recover and thrive after birth trauma or severe accident. After all, if things go badly, you can always change your mind.

A better approach to family members of very sick and apparently damaged newborns or adults is to be modest, saying: "Although I am as concerned as you are, I have seen patients just as sick who recover and some who ought to and don't. I can't know in which category your family member will be. I do know that negative prognostication can lead to the family giving up and withdrawing, whereas families who engage with their sick family member enhance recovery."

As a neonatologist in the 1970s, I shared other neonatologists' great skepticism about the future for the very small premature infants in our care. Neonatologist Saroj Saigal has followed very small infants who weighed in the range of eight hundred to a thousand grams at birth for an astonishing thirty years. She compared them to a matched sample of babies of normal birth weight.[1] Most of the tiny survivors live normal and productive lives, are married and have educational degrees. Some have minimal deficits and a few have severe deficits, but overall their quality of life as a group is comparable to the normal-weight newborns.

In her powerful book *Fallen*, Kara Stanley details the care her husband, Simon, received when he was in a deep coma after falling off a roof.[2] On arrival to hospital by air ambulance, Kara was exposed to the first of many negative comments. The trauma team gave a dismal prognosis, employing the Glasgow Coma Scale.

This scale is good for getting an idea of prognosis for a population of patients, but it may not be useful for individuals. Simon's result was 3.3, the lowest possible score.

After Simon's craniotomy, Kara received a relatively positive statement from one neurosurgeon: "The underlying tissue beneath the bleed looked good. There is room to hope." As this doctor spoke of hope, Kara remembers that his facial expression and body language conveyed anything but.

Soon after, a young neurosurgeon contradicted the senior neurosurgeon, saying: "Simon's brain injuries are global and diffuse. If he survives, it is impossible to predict which areas of the brain might be affected, possibly all of them. The bleeding in his brain is extensive, and blood is toxic to neurons. Wherever there is blood, neurons have died. The underlying tissue does not look good. His brain is soaked with blood, like soup with neurons swimming in it."

Other comments from physicians and nurses included:

- "His left pupil is blown."
- "Executive functions may well be lost."
- "Damage to the optic nerve may be permanent." (Within days his vision was normal.)
- "We are talking about the possibility that Simon might wind up in a long-term facility."
- "Simon's brain will never be as good as it was before."

But an ICU nurse said: "You spend days working with someone you are certain is hopeless. A few weeks later you meet them in the hospital hallways, awake and responsive. Then it all feels worthwhile."

Kara, who is a fine writer, never paid much attention to negative prognoses. She filtered them out and fully engaged with Simon, even when he was in a coma. Although Simon is now paraplegic, he has recovered full use of his upper body and his hands. He is fully engaged with his family and is a well-regarded guitar player and singer/composer. He lives a positive and productive life. Simon's recovery fit well with the many experiences that had shown me the importance of prognostic modesty in medicine.

As a medical student returning to finish my last year at Stanford medical school, I still had some elective time left. I took a six-week elective in the newborn intensive care unit. One of my responsibilities, which meant I was regularly on duty alone overnight, was to be in charge of premature infants in various states of illness. This was perhaps the first of a series of assignments where, because of my Ethiopian experience, faculty would give me more responsibility than was usual for a medical student or resident. Although I had "lost" a year from medical school while in Ethiopia, I was regularly promoted or advanced to positions of more responsibility, such that I did not lose any time at all.

In 1965, premature infants with hyaline membrane disease, called respiratory distress syndrome (RDS), were for the first time being supported with respirators. At Stanford, on Dr. Sunshine's newborn unit, we adapted adult respirators for the purpose but only for the sickest. There were many problems with equipment that was designed for adults. We knew that the respirator tubing was too long for such small infants, whose weight was generally in the range of 1,200 to 1,700 grams. As well, the equipment was not sensitive enough for the task. But we did what we could. Neonatology was just developing as a specialty in those days. As the results were so poor with those early devices, most neonatologists resisted the use of respirators.

On duty one night, I became increasingly concerned about the well-being of one premature infant in respiratory distress. His condition was deteriorating. It was becoming more and more difficult for me to maintain the infant's oxygen level. I had reached the limit of what the respirator could do. Knowing that I needed help, I looked on the list of covering attending physicians. At about 3 a.m. I called Dr. Marshall Klaus. I had never met him. Dr. Klaus arrived in good time and examined the infant and studied the blood oxygen results. Expecting some help, I was stunned to hear him say: "What do you think this baby is thinking?" I don't remember exactly what I said, but I might have been a bit rude.

Dr. Klaus then said: "How do you think this baby's mother felt when she had to go home and leave her baby behind?" I am sure that my response was less than positive. But I do remember vividly what he next said: "Mr. Klein, this baby is going to die and there is nothing further that we can do for him. Let's think about what we can do to help his unfortunate mother."

I could not relate to Dr. Klaus. I was still in cure mode. Dr. Klaus was looking at the big picture. At the time, I didn't know that he was deeply involved with Dr. John Kennell in the care of premature infants, and he was about to publish one of the first studies on maternal-infant bonding. Developmentally, I was not in a mindset to appreciate Dr. Klaus, but it was not too many years later that I was consulting him regularly. He became one of my key mentors, a relationship that continued until his death in 2017 in his early nineties.

14. OBSTETRICS COMES BACK TO BITE ME

IT WAS THE FIRST DAY of one of my remaining clerkships: an obstetrics and gynecology rotation at Stanford Hospital. Following the usual pattern, I was attending births with supervision. I had completed a couple when I felt a firm hand on my shoulder. It was the professor and university chair of obstetrics and gynecology.

His face red, he hissed: "Come into my office, Mr. Klein."

I followed, ignorant of the reason for the invitation. I had not met him before. His office was decorated with pictures of his teachers and men in beards, and various lethal-looking instruments.

After a long silence, he said: "On my service, every woman will receive an episiotomy. And if she does not get one before the birth, she will get one after." The last part of his statement must have been a sick joke, or at least I hope it was a joke: "If you want to practise primitive medicine, you will have to go to the county hospital."

My crime? I was delivering babies without episiotomy (and usually without tears), just as the Ethiopian midwives had taught me. I never thought I was doing anything abnormal. He indeed exiled me to the Santa Clara county hospital. In US medicine, then and even today, the county hospital generally provides free medical treatment for poor people. The residents run the show, with attending physicians rarely on the scene.

With some trepidation, I presented myself to the chief resident in OB/GYN at the county hospital, carrying a sealed envelope. I don't know what the letter inside said, presumably something negative. Looking bored, he glanced at the letter, looked up from his desk and said: "So what do you want to do while you are here?" I remember mumbling something inane like: "I'd like to deliver babies and study obstetrics and gynecology." To which he replied: "Anything else?" My reply was perhaps prophetic: "How about me looking after the babies after I deliver them?" Based on my experience in Ethiopia, it seemed a natural thing to request.

The chief resident was not troubled by my reply, merely stating: "You will have to talk about that with the chief of pediatrics." At that time and still today, everything was organized in silos. So I presented myself to the chief of pediatrics, a respected physician who later became one of the heads of pediatrics at Stanford Hospital. When I arrived at the office of Gordon Williams, I saw that I was meeting a man who had overcome much. He had been born with a congenital malformation that I happened to recognize. He was very short and had a large head with a prominent forehead and clubbed feet. He walked with two canes. And I knew that he had treated hydrocephalus. These are all consequences of a congenital syndrome known as the Arnold-Chiari malformation, in which there is a block in spinal fluid circulation at the base of the skull. For Dr. Williams to have survived intact, a neurosurgeon must have performed a shunt to lower the pressure in the cavities of his brain to arrest the hydrocephalus and drain off the spinal fluid. Otherwise, the pressure would have built up and prevented the normal development of his brain.

After presenting my proposal, he said: "Mr. Klein, that's a great idea. Why don't you do that?" In retrospect, I had no name for what I was doing, having never seen a GP during my education at Stanford, and in 1965–66, academic family medicine had not yet been invented in the US or Canada. Most general practitioners took a one-year rotating internship and just started practising, learning on the job, as their training never included office-based practice. Their education consisted of rotating through the major hospital-based specialties, often spending time on esoteric diseases that they would never see, certainly not in the context of an ambulatory patient. If you have never seen a family doctor, it is hard to imagine being one. We have a joke in family practice education. What are the three principles of teaching family practice? The first is *role models*. The second is *role models*. The third is *role models*. There are no other principles.

Because of the flexibility of the staff at the county hospital, I had a wonderful experience delivering babies and caring for them in my own personal family practice program in maternal and child health. The early experience working with midwives in Ethiopia and then my short career on the OB/GYN clerkship at the county hospital greatly influenced my later practice and research, but it took many years for me to realize to what extent.

From a technical point of view, I had a good educational experience working at the county hospital. But I was nevertheless acutely aware that I was exposed to, and benefitting from, the worst of US medicine—a structure that continues to this day, despite minor attempts to rectify it, such as the Affordable Care Act (Obamacare) and even the phony attempts at replacement or reform in 2017 by the Trump administration and the Republican-dominated Congress and Senate. In 1960, as a first-year medical student, the awareness of the need to improve the health care system had already led me to join the Student American Medical Association. Working with fellow students, I fought for a single-payer system, much like what exists in Canada. We campaigned for legislation then known as the King-Anderson Bill, which of course failed. Hard to believe that the US is still struggling with this issue, with organized medicine, big pharma and the insurance industry perpetually successful in blocking the implementation of what the country desperately needs.

Many medical students are really radical as they begin their training. These ideals get beaten out of them as they go on with their education. From the vantage point of working and living in Canada, I continue to be amazed at how the American public has been bamboozled into believing that what they really need is bad for them. They have been led to believe in their "freedom" to suffer and become destitute and wind up on welfare after a major illness leads to family bankruptcy. But Canadians ought not feel complacent. American multinational companies are knocking at our door to try to gain access to a lucrative market.

MY NEW CLASS

Because I had spent a year and a half in Ethiopia, when I returned I was a member of the following class. I had missed the joy of graduating with the classmates who had helped me get through those difficult preclinical years.

But returning to a new class was in some ways a gift, as I got to meet a whole other group of students, and because of my separation and divorce, I was in a more open state to interact with others. Plus, my old buddy Arthur was now one of my classmates.

Arthur Zelman and I had met before medical school, through my college roommate David Sigman. Both had gone to high school in Forest Hills, New York. Arthur and I shared some leftish politics and a relatively radical view of the place of medicine in society. We both saw medicine as a calling and an opportunity to assist communities less fortunate to improve their lives. Arthur was a good guitar player, and playing folk songs and singing along was a favourite activity. I next got to see Arthur when he was just beginning medical school. As every student had to have their own microscope, to earn a little money I became a microscope salesman. I remember how impressed Arthur was with my entrepreneurial spirit. In fact, this was the last time I can remember being entrepreneurial. I was a big-deal second-year student when Arthur arrived in his broken-down car with his pal Luke. The car had no muffler, as far as I could tell, and Luke was holding the door closed on the passenger side.

Now classmates, Arthur and I happened to begin one of our surgical rotations together. Keen, we arrived in the surgical dressing area early and got dressed in "greens." Surgeons were coming in and out of the locker area and chatting around the coffee machine. We were both aware that little or nothing was being said about the surgical cases. The staff surgeons were discussing their financial woes, their stocks and their conservative politics. Suddenly, Arthur got up, theatrically stripped off his surgical scrubs and bellowed, "If this is what medicine is all about, I want nothing to do with it!" And he left. He really left—medical school. I was worried. It looked like he was actually never going to become a physician, and I was losing a friend in the program.

But I was wrong. After a short time away from medicine, Arthur was working at the Palo Alto veterans hospital. This was a sprawling multi-building complex made famous by the film *One Flew Over the Cuckoo's Nest*, which was shot there. We all knew a Nurse Ratched type who berated us. We medical students received part of our psychiatric education there, largely learning from veterans of the Korean War. In most cases, the vets had joined up with the Marines. Many had a romantic notion of the war as the crucible of their manhood. What we saw were broken men who were alcoholic, drug dependent and depressed.

Many had what was later called post-traumatic stress disorder (PTSD), though in the 1960s no such term was in use by mental health professionals. In World War I it was called shell shock.

A mainstay of the psychiatric treatment at the VA hospital was group therapy, beginning every morning with a group circle, led by a psychiatrist faculty member. The patients would tell their story or make other contributions, followed by criticism from the other patients, then questions and some commentary by the psychiatrist ward leader. I had experienced the same process early in my training at the VA. What seemed clear to me was that few patients got better, and it seemed like nobody ever left. Arthur must have felt the same, as rather than sitting around in a circle, he formed a company with the patients and sold their services in the community as house painters.

Wonder of wonders, Arthur's patients generally got better and were often permanently discharged. After a year of running this company, helping the patients get back on their feet and making some money in the process, Arthur rejoined Stanford medical school, now a year behind me.

Arthur's story triggered a memory of my own student psychiatry rotation at the same VA hospital. I was following the usual educational pattern, taking part in the therapeutic circle, when one of the patients accused me of being attracted to him. Although I was flustered inside, externally I kept my cool and simply said that he must have misinterpreted my interest in his well-being as a homosexual interest. The other patients, several of whom were struggling with homosexual issues, thought that I was so cool and calm that it solidified my role as a student shrink. In their therapeutic society, such accusations generally led to fighting.

During that same rotation, the psychiatrist in charge of the ward assigned me a patient who had been in the Women's Army Corps for a long time and had suffered what used to be called "a breakdown." My job was to talk with her every day in a "therapeutic relationship," whatever that was for a fourth-year student. As the hospital was stuffy and spartan and the sun was shining outside, I decided to listen to her story while we walked the manicured grounds. This I did for more than a week, strolling the grounds, attentively listening to her sad life story. Since I did not really know what to do to help her, I just listened and commiserated.

If, in the opinion of the ward psychiatrist, it was safe enough, the patients could be granted leave over weekends. So one Friday afternoon, my patient was granted leave to visit her family in San Francisco. I was pleased that the psychiatrist felt that she had improved enough to allow this privilege. But come Monday morning she had not returned. I was pleased that the patient felt well enough to stay away longer. The psychiatrist felt otherwise. "Mr. Klein, I don't know what you did to her, but if your patient has committed suicide, it is your fault." I was terrified. I was convinced that I must indeed have done something wrong. I skipped lunch and dinner and went home, certain that she had killed herself.

However, on Tuesday morning, during our usual circle meeting, the patient waltzed in, looking cheerful and in good shape psychologically, according to my untrained eye. Without preamble, she blurted out that she felt it was time for her to be discharged. The psychiatrist was furious, saying in front of my student colleagues that I had ruined a therapeutic relationship that he had been building for many weeks.

I doubt that I had anything to do with the patient's seeming improvement, but boy was I pissed. After recovering from the terror engendered by the psychiatrist's accusations, I realized the psychiatrist was way out of line. I went to the dean and complained. The dean called in the psychiatrist for a reprimand, stating that he had been guilty of abuse of power.

15. INTERNSHIP AT ALBERT EINSTEIN COLLEGE OF MEDICINE IN NEW YORK

ALTHOUGH MISSING MY DAUGHTER, MISHA, was heartbreaking, I thoroughly enjoyed my return to Stanford and made the most of both the training and my social relationships with the new class. Finishing Stanford medical school in June 1966, I was accepted as a pediatric intern at Albert Einstein College of Medicine and the Bronx Municipal Hospital Center, a New York City hospital serving a mixed poor and affluent community. In short order it became clear to my supervisors that once again my Ethiopian experience put me in a position to receive increased responsibility, especially on the infectious disease ward. The head of the pediatric service was Dr. Lewis Fraad, a thoughtful, supportive professor with whom I immediately connected. He was open and available and became another mentor.

Dr. Fraad and the department as a whole were strongly against the Vietnam War, which helped solidify my respect for them. I used some of my very limited off hours to work with doctors who were planning to oppose the war. My opposition to the war was enhanced by the knowledge that we all would be drafted into the Medical Corps immediately after internship, unless we had made other arrangements, such as getting into the US Public Health Service (USPHS). Joining the USPHS was an attractive alternative, as it not only kept you out of the military, but you could also learn some valuable skills that could be useful for your career. Some physicians, in return for a promise to serve the military after completing their specialist training, were allowed to continue their residency training. This second route was attractive, and many took it.

For several months during that internship year I was assigned to the Lincoln Hospital pediatric service. Lincoln Hospital was located in the Southeast Bronx, a virtual war zone. The hospital was understaffed and unbelievably rundown, so it was not unusual for the interns and residents to have to feed children and assist the nurses in diaper changing and general support. The neighbourhood was so dangerous that the interns and residents had to escort the nurses to the bus stop and stand with them until they were safely on the bus.

The diseases of the Lincoln Hospital children resembled those I had seen in Ethiopia: TB, meningitis, malnutrition and lots of lead poisoning, the latter a result of eating lead-based paint in the rundown tenements. A municipal hospital, it was run by interns and residents, under the supervision of Dr. Arnold Einhorn, an enigmatic but devoted pediatrician who gave us great responsibility.

"IF YOU LEAVE HER, I'LL KILL YOU"

Marisol was a three-year-old of Puerto Rican extraction. When she was well she seemed perfectly normal, but at regular intervals she would present in a semi-comatose state with dehydration and depressed respiration. Her lab work showed remarkably severe acidosis that was unresponsive to massive doses of bicarbonate. She was like a bottomless pit. No matter how we tried to correct her metabolic state, the acidosis returned, until finally, with time, it self-corrected. In the meantime, all we could do was keep her on a ventilator and wait.

One night at about 3 a.m., as I was running the ventilator and doing my best to keep her alive, her father approached me. He drew a gun and presented me with a twenty-dollar bill, stating, "Take the money. If you leave her, I'll kill you." I tried to explain in Spanish that I had no intention of leaving Marisol, and that money would make no difference. He became agitated. "Take the money or else." I took the money and days later when Marisol had stabilized I gave it back.

I did not know what was wrong with Marisol, but I suspected a rare form of genetically determined vitamin-dependent organic acidemia. No one at

Einstein had an answer. I later learned that during one of her recurrent episodes Marisol had died. A frozen sample of her blood finally confirmed the diagnosis of an obscure, untreatable genetic organic acidemia.

A PREMATURE INFANT: WRONG FLOOR

Lincoln was such an ancient and crumbling hospital that physical conditions were not ideal. Case in point: the delivery room and the pediatric service were on different floors. On this particular night, the elevators, as was often the case, were not functioning. I was called to the birth of a small premature infant. Standing at the elevator, with the baby in a transport isolette, I waited as long as I could. Finally, I wrapped the infant in a blanket, opened my shirt, held the baby against my bare chest and ran down the back stairs to the pediatric ward, where fortunately, the baby did well.

EDDIE B.

When I was on duty in the hospital emergency room in the middle of the night (smoking a pipe, I might add—and no one said a word in those days) a Black mother appeared with her son of about eight years old. Gravely, she said: "He has convulsions, rheumatic fever and 'sickly' cell disease."

I was duly impressed and admitted him. During the course of a week of investigations I determined that he had none of those diseases. He was healthy. The reality was that the mother was holding down two jobs and needed Eddie to be at home from school caring for his two younger siblings.

I finally figured out that I was dealing with the rare Munchausen's syndrome by proxy. In this condition, a third party, usually a parent, finds it in his or her interest for someone else to be sick. Did she really think Eddie had all those diseases? Yes, she did. She really believed that he was as sick as she had described. She actually needed Eddie to have these diseases.

What about school? Working with a social worker, I found out that Eddie was enrolled in schools in both Brooklyn and the Bronx. As far as I could tell, he had missed 70 per cent of the days in the Bronx school, and he had not attended the Brooklyn school at all—yet he was advanced grade to grade in both. When I called one of the principals with this incredible story and asked why he had passed, the principal actually said: "He never made any trouble." Getting Eddie sorted out was a major undertaking, and I am not sure that we ever really succeeded.

JUST A ROUTINE PRE-OP PHYSICAL

These kinds of quirky things don't happen just to poor inner-city kids. On duty at the upscale Einstein College hospital, I was admitting a young boy for a routine hernia operation the next day. The mother arrived with a box full of medications for his asthma and began to list for me the detailed schedule of medications to be employed: "You give him this pill at 4 p.m., these two at six, this inhaler at eight," et cetera.

I listened attentively. Then I listened to his chest. It was perfect, pristine. I shared my observation with his mother—perfect lungs. Not a wheeze in evidence.

"Dr. Klein, that is the way it always starts."

ASTHMA—OF SORTS

Another of my young patients, with what at first appeared to be a refractory case of asthma, also demonstrated the strange ways that illness can present. The boy's father was a taxi driver, who rarely saw the boy—except when the boy was sick. The son "needed" to have an attack to see his dad. Whenever he had an attack, he would call his father, who would arrive in his taxi and off they would go to the emergency room, where they would have a more or less pleasant evening together. I arranged for regular social meetings of the father and son. The emergency visits largely stopped.

DIABETES IN A PRETEEN

While caring for an eleven-year-old diabetic who required insulin, I found it was difficult to encourage him to keep a record of his urine test results. At last, one day he proudly presented his record book. On careful perusal, I saw that it detailed his test results for the next six months.

16. NEW LOVE

During my internship at Einstein my social life was pretty non-existent. I was on duty every other night and usually so tired on my night off that I was pretty useless. As 1966 was turning into 1967, I looked around for a nice midwinter vacation. As was our pattern, my daughter, Misha, arrived by plane from Portland for the start of our vacation. A friend from the original class in medical school, Bob Erickson, and his wife, Sandy, were planning a camping trip to the US Virgin Islands with their two kids and invited Misha and me to come along. Great news, except that it turned out that the Ericksons had another friend, Bonnie Sherr, who had planned a trip to Spain but had suddenly realized that her passport had expired. The Ericksons invited her along too. I was annoyed. It looked like a setup, a two-week blind date. But what could I do?

Then it turned out that another medical school friend, Howard Fields, was getting married on New Year's Eve. He and Carol had no firm honeymoon plans so they came along too. Misha fell in love with Bonnie at the airport and they read *Are You My Mother?* on the airplane. It was the '60s and there was lots of smoking pot. Howard thought he was a fish and had to be rescued. Swimming amid ocean phosphorescence, under the romantic influence of the smoke and the tropical air, Bonnie and I became a couple almost right away, outdoing the newlyweds. Bonnie claims that she was hooked when she saw me carrying my Ethiopian Airlines bag, but I don't believe it.

Despite having shared a wonderful two-week fling, neither of us knew whether we would see each other again. But soon after, we were dating. An anti-war activist herself, Bonnie became very much a part of the evolving plans for what to do about the war. I also admired her commitment to social justice. In her teens, Bonnie had been a freedom rider and later a volunteer in Ghana. What was different and surprising was that, unlike my background, Bonnie's family was very conservative and uncritical of US policy. Somehow Bonnie had moved beyond her family values to become a thoughtful, politically astute woman who acted upon her beliefs. She went to Barnard College in New York City, had studied acting at Carnegie Mellon University in Pittsburgh and, at the time we met, she was a graduate from the MA documentary film program at Stanford and was freelancing in New York City. I admired Bonnie's openness and the way that she immediately connected with Misha, and I fell for her playful, relaxed yet serious demeanour.

Before Bonnie and I began our romantic relationship, before my pediatric internship had started and even before I finished medical school, world events were unfolding that would forever shape our lives. My anti-war activities and my life as a "red diaper baby" would finally surface in the context of my dealings with the US Army.

17. DR. MICHAEL KLEIN VERSUS THE US ARMY

ON NOVEMBER 22, 1963, PRESIDENT John F. Kennedy was assassinated. Like many others, I vividly remember where I was when it happened. I was a third-year medical student on the pediatric floor, helping look after a child with an obscure disease. There was a TV above her crib, and the news flashed on the screen. Throughout the hospital, on all the wards, staff stopped what they were doing and leaned over patients' beds to receive the terrible news. Most were crying. We had begun to be proud of our country. The Peace Corps had been founded and young people were engaged. We thought we could change the world. The medical community was no different.

In the two years that Kennedy was president, we thought he was masterful in avoiding nuclear war in the Cuban Missile Crisis. These were heady days. We knew little about the evolving Vietnam War, but US involvement was thought to be limited. That changed with the escalation in 1964, and when regular US combat units were deployed at the beginning of 1965—just in time for us med students to start worrying about what branch of medicine we would select for future training.

For some of us, that foolish and unjust war attracted us to the protest movement. When some of my medical student friends and I, with Dr. Greenberg, marched against the war, our FBI files were probably started, though I later learned mine had begun earlier. I was ready to serve my country in any number of alternative humanitarian ways but not as part of the Vietnam War effort. During the war, students had ways of avoiding the draft: get married, get a college deferment or, if inventive, fake an illness. Most of these alternatives were not available to poor kids, who were disproportionally from minorities. Off went poor kids from the inner cities and depressed rural areas to fight a rich man's war, while rich kids could find a way to avoid military service. A good example is Donald Trump's bogus heel spurs. Rich kids could find a cooperative doctor to assert whatever... Trump can't even remember which side had the spur, and spurs don't go away without treatment. Later, when a lottery was in effect, you could get lucky and receive a high number, thus guaranteeing a reprieve. But none of this applied to physicians. In one way or another, we all got drafted.

I preferred the option of joining the United States Public Health Service (USPHS), but I was also exploring applying to my draft board as a conscientious objector (CO). The idea of being a physician CO was difficult for many to understand. "What's the problem? You're not going to be asked to kill anybody." True, but the Uniform Code of Military Justice, the law that governs all persons and all roles in the US military, is clear: a military physician's "primary responsibility is to support the mission." Specifically, the duty of the military physician is to return the soldier to combat or his usual role, not to address the soldier's well-being. Consequently, many soldiers were being returned to their units in a less than ideal shape, both medically and psychologically. Many deeply damaged soldiers were dealing with their stress through heavy use of alcohol and illicit drugs.

All I knew was that I wanted nothing to do with the military. So in the spring of 1966, while I was finishing medical school at Stanford, and about to enter my pediatric internship in New York, I began intensive work on ways to avoid the military. I followed two parallel paths: I applied to the USPHS, and I also applied to my local draft board as a CO.

Apart from my feelings about being part of the military, I had specific and fundamental issues with the US involvement in the Vietnam War. I was willing to serve my country but not in an essentially local national struggle. Post–World War II, most Americans saw the French as colonial occupiers in Vietnam and supported emerging anti-colonial nationalism—that was, until the start of the Cold War and McCarthyism of the 1950s and the Korean War.

Although he had been discredited, in the 1960s McCarthy's influence was still at play. Many of the members of the US administrations under Kennedy and then Johnson were virulently anti-communist. Inside the US government itself it was clear that those who saw Vietnam as an internal fight between nationalists and a corrupt puppet regime, rather than communism versus freedom, found their positions and future in jeopardy. This was true also of the military leaders, many of whom thought the US ought to leave Vietnam alone. Holding that position led them to being sidelined by overly optimistic Joint Chiefs of Staff and the gung-ho military leadership based in Vietnam—who somehow managed to see losses as victories and sometimes even altered negative assessments by their own staff, censoring reports of disastrous US battle outcomes. Sanitized reports from the military leadership even kept US presidents in the dark about the reality on the ground.

Smarting from the "loss of China" to the communists, the leaders in the White House convinced themselves that the domino theory applied—that if Vietnam fell, it was the beginning of the end for all of Southeast Asia. The White House did not appreciate that all communism was not the same, that Vietnam was neither the Soviet Union nor China. My draft board was of the same mind, the goal being to defeat communism at all costs. Fully aware of this history and the inexorable pursuit of the war, there was no way that I was going to serve in Vietnam—a bogus, illegal, immoral, phony, unwinnable war. Our leaders failed to grasp that this was a war between a corrupt dictatorship in the south and a popular anti-colonial nationalist insurrection driven by the north.

In preparing my CO application, I consulted widely. I collected letters of support from teachers and respected people in society. As CO status is dependent on deeply held religious beliefs, I consulted with a rabbi sympathetic to my views on the Vietnam War. Rabbi Robert E. Goldburg was extremely helpful in teaching me about the Biblical and Torah sources that would support my position. He was a long-serving rabbi, whose Hamden, Connecticut, congregation was the longest continuous Jewish congregation in the US.

Rabbi Goldburg was an obvious choice to help me prepare my CO application. Apart from his opposition to the Vietnam War, he was outspoken in his support of civil rights and other causes. During his rabbinate, he often invited guest speakers who were considered controversial, like Dr. Daniel Ellsberg and Stokely Carmichael. The Reverend Dr. Martin Luther King Jr. preached at Rabbi Goldburg's synagogue, Mishkan Israel, in 1961. Rabbi Goldburg had spoken out against McCarthyism and the HUAC when it subpoenaed writers and artists to investigate their political attitudes. His sermons emphasized the harmony between Jewish values and democratic principles, weaving together themes from the Talmud, Shakespeare and contemporary writers. I could relate to this Judaism, and it allowed me to address some of the religious questions in the CO document. But it was obvious that for me to be a legitimate CO was a stretch. To be clear, I would have served in the military in World War II. I was no Quaker.

My beliefs were based on the "brotherhood of man" (sexist words, used then) and the inability of war to distinguish who is "worthy to die." In early drafts of my CO application, I used many sections from the Old Testament to support my religious convictions, but in the end I found that this was disingenuous, as I was not a conventionally religious person. Hence, I cut almost all this extensive religious material out of the final document.

I knew I was pushing the conventional definitions of being a CO, so instead, as a pediatrician-in-training, I spoke in the application to the particular vulnerability of children as the innocent victims of war, explored war as based primarily on imbalances in wealth and named preventive medicine as a much-preferred way to avoid both poverty and war. I explained my belief that the military physician was just as much an instrument of war as the soldier. I expressed my willingness to serve my country in an alternative way, unconnected to war. I cited my stints in Mexico and Ethiopia as support for my views and actions. I detailed my public presentations and writings on these experiences. I indicated that I could best serve my country in the USPHS or in a similar situation where my personal principles and religious views would not be in conflict. My application was supported by letters from my high school history teacher, the dean of medicine at Stanford, a very religious professor of public health and preventive medicine at Stanford, my supervising professors at Albert Einstein and Rabbi Goldburg.

In 1967, just prior to my CO hearing at my local draft board, I wrote the board in detail about my support for another physician who had run afoul of the military, Dr. Howard Levy. I and hundreds of other physicians had signed an open letter in the *New York Times* supporting Dr. Levy, who was sent to military prison for refusing to obey orders to teach medical corpsmen skills that would be used for political purposes. "The medical art of healing," he said, "was becoming the handmaiden of political objectives."

My CO application clearly outlined exactly what I would be facing were I to join the military. I, too, would have disobeyed such an order that employed medicine as a tool to bring the Vietnamese people over to the US side in what was called the Pacification Campaign. The plan was to bribe poor, often sick villagers by offering them medical treatment. Like Levy, I felt that such an order violated the Hippocratic oath. Dr. Levy found his personal and medical ethics conflicted with his role as a military physician. But in doing so, Dr. Levy failed to support the mission, and he was court-martialled. The powerful poster of a mild-mannered Dr. Levy being led away in handcuffs to be imprisoned at Fort Leavenworth for two and a half years was on my wall for many years as a reminder of his principled stance and the price he paid. Our son, Seth, has his own framed copy on his living room wall. The poster ironically proclaimed, *Join the New Action Army*.

In May 2016, I managed to track down Dr. Howard Levy. In his eighties, he is still a New York dermatologist, still practising at Lincoln Hospital, where I had trained during my internship at Albert Einstein. His politics, commitment to his patients and social conscience remain intact.

My hearing before my draft board was an unpleasant seventeen-minute interview with four hostile, sullen board members. They did not allow me any time to develop my position. It was obvious that they had not read my file. They focused on how it is impossible for a physician to be a CO, employing the usual argument that they were not asking me to shoot anyone. My CO application and later appeal were quickly denied, followed rapidly by a change in my draft status from the student deferment of 2-S to 1-A, or "available for unrestricted military service."

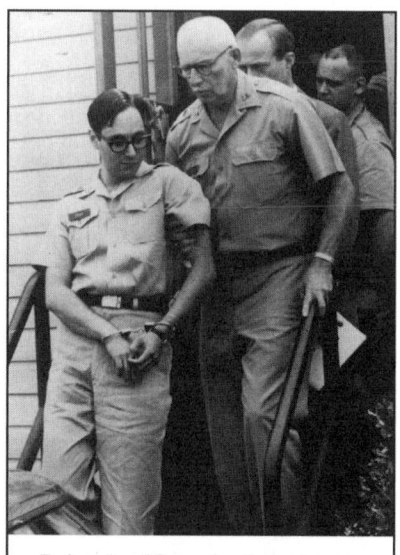

Join the New Action Army

Dr. Howard Levy in 1967, being led away in handcuffs to serve two and a half years in military prison for refusing to train Green Beret army medics. Photo courtesy of Howard Levy

The good news was that on August 23, 1966, I received a letter from the USPHS and US National Institutes of Health (NIH), indicating I had been successful in finding an acceptable alternative to the military that would allow me to serve my country in a way that fit my values. Specifically, the National Institute of Neurological Diseases and Blindness outlined a plan for me to enter the USPHS in the field of perinatal epidemiology at the NIH and the Communicable Disease Center in Atlanta, Georgia.

It was a huge relief. They were interested in training me in the very area of my interest. Problem solved. This would have fit perfectly with what would become my future major clinical and research interests. I immediately called to accept the offer.

I didn't know at the time but learned later through a Freedom of Information request that shortly after my acceptance into the USPHS, the USPHS sent a routine letter to my draft board inquiring about my status. The board replied: "He is a conscientious objector." In point of fact, I was only *an applicant* for conscientious objector status. Based on this reply from the draft board, in September a critical letter followed from the USPHS to me and my draft board that withdrew the offer of a position as a future USPHS commissioned officer.

It turns out that in times of national emergency the USPHS could be activated as a quasi-military force, and its officers could be loaned to any branch of the US military. Being a CO was actually incompatible with being an officer in the USPHS. If I had known this, I would have withdrawn my application for CO status, and my appointment to the USPHS would have gone ahead successfully.

My draft board did not lose any time. Within days of receiving the reply from the USPHS that cancelled my appointment, they ordered me to report for an armed forces physical examination. As part of the rapidly evolving process, I was required to fill out a form in advance of my physical that listed my previous employments and asked, among other questions, if I was ever a member of the Communist Party. I checked no.

In October 1966, I reported for my army physical exam, in a huge building that processed hundreds of inductees every day. It was organized into stations—urine processing, hearing testing, X-ray, chest exam, rectal exam, et cetera. Each station was manned by a uniformed army medical corpsman, except for the physical exam stations, which were run by army medical doctors.

I could not help thinking that the setup sounded just like Arlo Guthrie's famous "Alice's Restaurant" anthem. In fact, Guthrie was examined in the very same New York building and later rejected for military service.

We doctors were processed as a separate group. At each station, the doctors were identified and brought to the head of the line. This was usually accompanied by protests and occasional booing from the regular inductees, who were generally Black or Puerto Rican and obviously poor. The doctors were all white.

First we had our urine tested, then headed into soundproof audiology booths for a hearing test. At the end of my session the corpsman approached me, hand extended: "Shake, doc. You are one in a million. You could hear a flea pissing on cotton at a hundred yards." I was so proud. Some of the inductees were trying to fake an audiogram, but the signals were delivered randomly and it was obvious when someone was faking. I did not want to enter the army, but I was not going to get out by faking an audiogram.

At the final station I was required to fill out a lengthy form known as the Attorney General's List, a list of presumed communist or communist front organizations. I did not sign the form to indicate I had not been a member of any of these organizations, though some sounded vaguely familiar. I did indicate I was a member of the National Association for the Advancement of Colored People (NAACP), the Committee for a Sane Nuclear Policy (SANE) and the American Civil Liberties Union (ACLU). The form asked if I had ever been in the employ of a foreign power. I checked yes, as I had been employed by the Ethiopian government. But I did not elaborate.

Another section of the form required that I select one of the armed services as my preference. I checked none of the boxes for army, navy, or air force. Below I wrote: "I am a conscientious objector. I will not serve in any branch. I will apply for CO status immediately on induction." When the corpsman studied the form, he was irate and told me that I needed to check one of the boxes. I refused. Again, he asked me to check one of the boxes. Again, I refused. After a few minutes, an imposing officer with lots of gold braid on his uniform appeared. He identified himself as a military psychiatrist and told me, "Son, you are making a huge mistake. You are in the process of ruining your life. You will never be able to practise medicine. Do yourself a favour, son, and check one of the boxes."

I replied that as I was not in the military, I didn't have to. I turned my back on him, and a bit shaken, I left the officer standing there and returned to the hospital to resume my duties.

Shortly thereafter, I was notified that I was to be interviewed by US Army Intelligence about my CO application, my employment by the Ethiopian Ministry of Health and my failure to choose a military service. I quickly made an appointment with John Somers, a young lawyer in a prestigious New York law firm. He was providing pro bono legal support for a variety of war resistors. I was his only physician client, his usual client being a poor draftee from the inner city. I learned years later that he was a member of the Catholic Worker Movement, an organization that requires 40 per cent pro bono work from its members.

About the same time, I moved in with Bonnie. Our relationship was serious, but we were not talking about marriage. We had an apartment in Chelsea on the Lower West Side of New York. I commuted up either the west side or east side highway to my internship in the Bronx. I was on duty every second or third night and slept in the hospital when on duty. My plan was to go to jail rather than serve in the military.

After much stalling on my part, claiming that the dates the army gave me for the interview conflicted with my on-call duties, my lawyer decided that we would eventually have to agree to the interview. Failing to be interviewed could result in my being considered non-compliant, with the consequence that I would be drafted, not as a doctor but as a foot soldier.

My lawyer's plan was that under questioning, I was to appear polite and fully cooperative. I would attempt to answer the questions in a forthright manner. He, however, would prevent me from answering most questions. Despite his normal mild manner and polite demeanour, for the interview, he would appear to be difficult, aggressive, unpleasant and uncooperative. This version of good cop/bad cop was designed to present me as a loyal American trying to be cooperative and my lawyer as someone with whom the army would not look forward to dealing.

We arrived for the first of three interviews and were ushered into a small airless, windowless cubicle, where Army Special Agents Gainey and Bellingham were seated. Then followed a negotiation between Mr. Somers and the agents, in which Mr. Somers demanded that a full transcript of the proceedings be created, made available for our records and signed off by all parties. The agents claimed that this was impossible, as there were no facilities or equipment available for such, and furthermore, the request was irregular—this was not done. Mr. Somers replied that unless his request was honoured, we were leaving. After much grumbling, the agents left to consult, returning to reiterate their position.

Mr. Somers happened to know shorthand and offered to create a record and have it typed out for mutual study and approval. Stunned, the agents reluctantly agreed. Mr. Somers wrote very rapidly in shorthand, while the agents laboriously wrote their versions in longhand. Mr. Somers would finish writing and sit quietly, while the agents finished theirs. Their irritation was palpable. Mr. Somers controlled the interview.

I was asked, "If inducted, would you perform your lawful duties?" To which I responded, "I will exhaust every avenue open to me under the law to establish my claim to exemption from military service as a CO. If unsuccessful, I will perform duties, provided such duties are compatible with my medical ethics." I expressed my loyalty and allegiance to the United States of America.

There were many questions about my presence at various gatherings, which took place when I was in high school and even earlier. Some sounded familiar, including meetings, singing events and performances by people like Pete Seeger or Paul Robeson, or merely singalongs in living rooms. It was apparent that informers were present at these gatherings, and some of these informers may even have been friends. The amount of money invested by the spooks to determine if little old me was a loyal American was incredible.

Then, unbelievably, in early August 1967, before the end of the security investigation, I received a notification that it had been determined that I was acceptable for military service, despite the fact that the security hearing was all about determining *if* I was a loyal American and *if* I was suitable to be an officer in the US military. Someone, somewhere had upstaged that process, the left hand not knowing what the right hand was doing. I was now considered a loyal American and suitable officer material.

When I received my notice of acceptability to the army it seemed obvious to my lawyer and myself that the last scheduled meeting of the army security investigation team had become irrelevant. Nevertheless, Mr. Somers and I kept our previously scheduled meeting with the two special agents. Notice of acceptability in hand, we walked into the hearing room and showed it to the army intelligence investigators. They were genuinely flabbergasted. They could not explain how such a notice was possible, since they had not yet determined *if* I was loyal or suitable officer material. Mr. Somers demanded a copy of the transcript of the investigation, as we all had agreed. The agents now claimed that this would not be possible, as the office had no facilities to copy the material. Mild-mannered Mr. Somers blew his top. It was all an act, of course, but he played his part well. He was loud and abusive, and accused them of lying. Then he spied a copy machine through a partially open door. He demanded that the agents live up to our agreement. They finally agreed to provide the summary. Appearing angry, we stormed out.

I received my dreaded induction notice on a Friday. Bonnie was out of town that weekend at the annual Flaherty documentary film seminar, which that year was in Harriman, New York, a couple of hours up the New York State Thruway from New York City. I quickly got myself off duty and drove up to the seminar to tell her the news and my decision to go to jail rather than enter the military.

At the seminar, Bonnie had just seen a CBC documentary called *The Mills of the Gods* by Beryl Fox. Ms. Fox had managed to secure a ride on a US helicopter to film the Vietnam War up close. The "mills" referred to the helicopter blades beating their rhythm of death. The film showed soldiers gaily throwing napalm canisters out the aircraft door to fall upon Vietnamese villagers. This Canadian film revealed what we knew to be the truth of the Vietnam War, a truth never seen on US media.

Inspired that such a film could be made by a Canadian woman and broadcast by a Canadian national agency, the now-pregnant Bonnie said: "You can go to jail if you wish, but we can make a life-affirming decision, get married and go to Canada instead." We immediately made plans to immigrate.

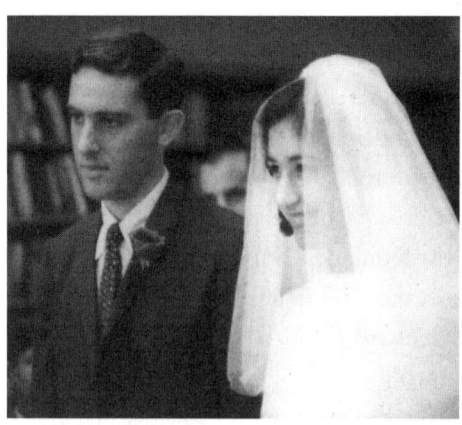

On August 19, 1967, Bonnie and I were hastily married in the office of Rabbi Goldburg. It was a small, strange ceremony attended by my parents, Anne and Philip Klein; Bonnie's parents, Nathan and Jennie Sherr; my brother, Henry, and his wife, Cecelia; Dr. Robert and Sandy Erickson (who had introduced us); Dr. Norma Zack, Bonnie's Barnard College roommate and best friend, who had come down from Boston; and Bonnie's sister, Razelle, and her

My marriage to Bonnie took place just before our immigration to Canada.

husband, William Frankl, a Philadelphia cardiologist. Dr. Frankl, my future brother-in-law, was particularly unhappy with the match. He told Bonnie that because of my political beliefs, I would never be able to practise medicine or make a living. He was also worried about the effect on Bonnie's father, who was in poor health. My parents approved of the marriage and knew of the plans that were to follow. Bonnie's did not approve. We celebrated our strange marriage with dinner at Howard Johnson's on the turnpike.

Our real wedding party took place several weeks later at my parents' house in Wanaque, New Jersey. It was a secret farewell party of friends and family, joyous for the most part, but only a very select few knew that we were shortly leaving the country, probably never to return.

As counselling draft evasion is a felony, my lawyer was not invited. He also advised us not to share anything of our plans, as people who knew could be found guilty of conspiring to aid draft evasion. There was a need for secrecy, especially given how porous I had learned friendships could be at the army security hearing. We drove to a public pay telephone for any important discussions rather than use the telephone in my parents' house. My parents' experience with the FBI and my father's being blacklisted during the McCarthy days added to our paranoia.

In preparation for our departure from the US, we had secretly consulted with the Montreal Council to Aid War Resisters, who advised that we would need to obtain immediate landed immigrant status to avoid being deported back to the US, where substantial jail time would result. The first priority was to secure a job offer from a Montreal hospital. To that end, I made a twenty-four-hour round trip to Montreal to meet with Professor Alan Ross, the chief of pediatrics at Montreal Children's Hospital. My mentor Bob Greenberg facilitated the link to Dr. Ross, through his colleague at Children's, Dr. Charles Scriver.

Based on my Ethiopian experience, and his personal position on the Vietnam War, Dr. Ross immediately offered me a senior residency position, which was a promotion, saving me a year of training time. He then provided a letter on McGill University and Montreal Children's Hospital stationery stating that I had a job.

On September 18, I filled out my papers to be a commissioned army officer and, as required, separately wrote to my draft board informing them that I had completed and mailed my commission papers. I was then an officer of the United States Army, awaiting my assignment.

As part of the application for a commission, which was to determine my precise military assignment, I detailed all the events relating to my CO application and parallel USPHS commission, which was rescinded because of the actions of my draft board. I wrote: "I plan to pursue my CO claim within the Armed Services. I want to make it perfectly clear that I am applying for this commission under duress and in order to avoid prosecution."

I then wrote to the army in detail about Dr. Howard Levy's case, stating "As a result of my continuing CO claim and the events which followed from the Levy affair, I find it necessary to state the following:

> I apply for a commission as an officer, but the Army must note and agree:
> 1. I will not serve in any combatant area such as Vietnam.
> 2. I will not be assigned duties which put me in a position where my ethical principles and religious and medical beliefs would be compromised. I have no desire to be another Captain Levy.
> 3. I will not obey orders which conflict with my personal, religious, or medical ethics or which violate the Hippocratic Oath."

I further reiterated that I found myself in this situation because my local draft board mishandled my case, causing me to lose my USPHS officer's commission. I made it clear that I would only accept a commission and an assignment if the above conditions and understandings were met in writing. Of course I knew that the army could never accept such conditions. I hoped, but did not expect, that the army would decide that I was more trouble than I was worth. This was the beginning of a series of deliberately contradictory and bizarre letters that I wrote to the army, asking what was taking them so long to give me my assignment. Tongue firmly planted in my cheek, I wrote: Yes, I was eager to serve, blah blah blah, but I repeatedly presented conditions that would be impossible for the army to accept.

On September 25, 1967, my draft board wrote to me again, stating that if I refused induction as an officer, I would be inducted as a foot soldier. The army again stated that my status then was as a United States military medical officer waiting for his assignment. Failing to report for duty would constitute being absent without leave (AWOL), or deserting, which would probably lead to long jail time.

The Montreal Council to Aid War Resistors told Bonnie and me that we should arrange to arrive in Montreal as our point of entry to Canada. Furthermore, we were strongly advised to arrive after midnight at Dorval airport, where we could expect to meet a French-Canadian immigration officer, as in those days the French Canadians had the less desirable night shift. The day shift would be English Canadians, many of whom had served in the Canadian military. They could be expected to be less sympathetic to an American deserter from the US military. In contrast, French Canadians were in general against conscription, especially "fighting for the queen." They were also likely to be against the Vietnam War. It was not at all clear that we would be welcomed, as the Canadian government had yet to instruct immigration officers to not ask questions about draft status.

Meanwhile, I had no way of knowing how the army was reacting to my deeply qualified commission papers. Was there a warrant out for my arrest? Had the Canadians been told to look out for me? We were anxious and paranoid, worried that I would be taken off the plane and returned to the army and jail.

We took only a suitcase each and boarded a flight to Montreal. Holding our breath, at 12:30 a.m. on October 2, 1967, our Air Canada flight arrived at Dorval airport. We joined the usual line of people entering Canada. As predicted, the immigration officer was a friendly French Canadian. We had brought current chest X-rays, as advised; our various diplomas; and, most importantly, the letter from Montreal Children's Hospital offering me a job. It was before the point system governed most immigration to Canada. The immigration officer on-site had great authority in deciding who would be admitted. Our officer effusively welcomed us to Canada. In twenty minutes we were landed immigrants, on the path to Canadian citizenship.

18. LIFE IN CANADA BEGINS

MONTREAL WAS EXUBERANT! IT WAS the time of Expo 67 and Montreal was the host. Bonnie and I went to as many of the innovative exhibits and films as possible. Bonnie spoke French and I enrolled in an intensive short-term French course. By mid-October I began my duties as a senior pediatric resident.

Apart from my job, for which I slept in the hospital every other night, I worked as a volunteer to help launch the Clinique des citoyens de Saint-Jacques, a free health clinic in a poor French neighbourhood in Montreal's East End. With McGill medical students Howard Bergman (now a professor and the head of family medicine at McGill) and Vania Jiménez (today director of professional and medical services for the Centre de santé et de services sociaux de la Montagne—a network of neighbourhood health care and social service clinics) and other Canadian health professionals, as well as other draft-resister physicians, we treated poor adults and children.

The clinic was a radical citizen-led enterprise that was using medicine as a political tool for community organizing. This did not mean that we used the patients. We were providing much-needed care in the pre-Medicare days. It was in that spirit that we ran a measles eradication campaign. The Institut Armand-Frappier in Montreal was developing a measles vaccine, but it was not yet available in Quebec. Meanwhile, measles was rampant and leading to serious illnesses in poor neighbourhoods. Something needed to be done. And who makes the vaccine in the US? The Dow Chemical Company, of course, the manufacturer of napalm, the weapon being used in Vietnam to burn villages and villagers and defoliate the countryside.

I swallowed my political pride and wrote to the Dow Chemical Company. We received several hundred vials of the measles vaccine, which we diluted to make them go further—after all, there are millions of virus particles in each vial, and the measles epidemic was serious business. Children were developing the complications of measles, including ear infections and bronchopneumonia, and a few were dying. The city was doing nothing. It felt like I was back in Chiapas.

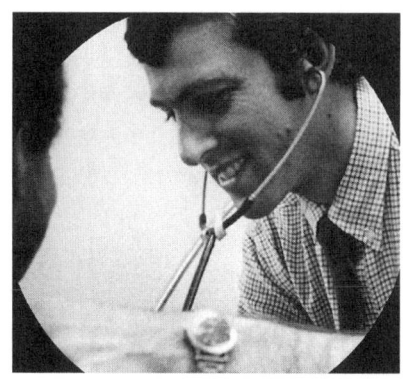

Examining a child at the Clinique des citoyens de Saint-Jacques, 1967.

We used our measles campaign to embarrass the City of Montreal into getting the needed vaccine, in the process using the measles story for community organizing. Bonnie, pregnant with Seth, made a film of our activities, *La clinique des citoyens/Citizens' Medicine*, which is still a landmark film, available from the National Film Board of Canada (NFB).

The staff at Montreal Children's Hospital could not have been more welcoming. They were generally opposed to the war, so they felt good about supporting their "draft dodger." I did not go into the details of my actual status as a deserter medical officer. Unlike me, Bonnie was able to commute to New York to finish some film work and then got her perfect job as an editor/director in the innovative Challenge for Change program at the NFB, where she made films about community organizing, including a series on Saul Alinsky, the famous American community organizer. Life was good.

We occasionally housed some draft evaders, and I corresponded with a group of medical students and residents in the US who were thinking of joining in a variety of actions, ranging from burning draft cards to leaving the US and continuing their medical studies in Canada. I was involved with the formation of a group called the Health Professionals Resistance Union. It was hard to know how many US physicians opposed the war, but I was told that there were more than one hundred physicians at the organizational meeting in Detroit. The big picture, however, was not about doctors and their resistance to the war. By various estimates, up to 200,000 Americans left for Canada as resisters, political refugees or just because they were ashamed of their country. More than half were women, some of whom came as spouses or partners, but many came alone because they could no longer live in a country pursuing an immoral and ultimately unwinnable war.

My parents could not have been more supportive, both emotionally and physically, much different from the families of many other draft evaders, some of whom were disowned. My parents rented a truck to bring our furniture. I was too busy in my job to think much about the reality that I might never cross the border to enter the US again.

Trying to remain within the letter, not the spirit, of the law, and following the army and draft board rules that required keeping them aware of your whereabouts, I immediately wrote to my draft board to tell them about my new address in Montreal. I again emphasized my schizoid eager hope that I would soon receive my assignment as an officer in the US Army Medical Corps. Specifically, I said: "What's taking the Army so long to use me as a medical officer?" I again emphasized that I would not obey orders that conflicted with my ethical principles and gave them a list of orders that I would not obey, knowing full well that they could not agree to such a position. I had no idea what my actual status might be. Was the army going to issue an arrest warrant or ask the Canadian government to deport me or just give up on me? I hoped the latter.

One Saturday morning in September, two young men dressed in dark business suits knocked on the door of our Montreal apartment. Bonnie and I were both at home. They showed us their identification as officers of the Royal Canadian Mounted Police.

One officer said, "We are here at the request of our colleagues in the FBI, who have requested that we verify if you are in Canada."

"As you can see, we are," I replied.

The RCMP officers, having fulfilled their role, left.

—:—

On April 24, 1968, Bonnie delivered Seth, eight pounds, thirteen ounces, at the Royal Victoria Hospital in Montreal. In those days, partners were not allowed in the delivery room. Photography was out of the question. I struggled to be present for the birth, even though I was a senior resident at the very hospital where the birth was taking place, and where I was the designated resuscitation officer with the responsibility of attending high-risk births and teaching resuscitation to the OB/GYN staff.

Breaking the rules of the day, Bonnie's obstetrician had agreed that I could be present. Unfortunately, he was not on call when Bonnie went into labour. Our obstetrician's covering partner did not share his openness. "I don't care what my partner agreed to. I won't have a physician-husband standing over my shoulder," he said. Bonnie held out until dawn, when her original physician arrived. Seth was delivered with the umbilical cord around his neck and a bit blue.

Dr. Robert Usher, my mentor in neonatology and by then a good friend, was paged. He cared for our newborn and brought baby Seth to the newborn ICU, where he almost didn't fit into the isolette designed for premature infants. But all was well. Dr. Usher was probably overcompensating, a known phenomenon where physicians get the best and worst care, often a combination of both.

Having arrived in Montreal under dramatic and frightening circumstances, nevertheless, we rapidly settled in. I loved my job as a senior resident. We had a new baby, and Bonnie had a dream job at the NFB. Then I finally received the news I was waiting for. In October 1968, a letter from the US Army stated I was "found not acceptable for induction under current standards" and thus not qualified for any military service. Shortly thereafter, I received a new classification from my draft board, a classification used for security risks and homosexuals. So now that I was a security risk and/or a homosexual, I could safely return to the United States without fear of arrest. All those wacky letters that I regularly wrote asking the army what was taking them so long to give me my assignment had apparently paid off. As I had hoped, the army must have decided that I was more trouble than I was worth. They did not need another Captain Levy.

I wrote to John Somers thanking him for all his help, expressing the belief that my family would not be leaving Canada for a long time, in part because I thought US employment or study would be unavailable to me. Mr. Somers was delighted to receive our update, as over many years I had stopped communicating with him for fear that his professional life might be compromised through associating with such a security risk.

Two years later, when Naomi was born, I was on staff at Royal Victoria Hospital, actually within the department of obstetrics and gynecology. I was looking forward to taking pictures of the birth. The chief nurse of what was called in those days the "Case Room" (what's a case?) saw me with a camera in the delivery and labour room. "Dr. Klein," she said, "Dr. Maugham [the chief of OB/GYN] does not allow the taking of pictures of birth."

"What?" I said. "It's my wife and child, and I work here."

She was adamant. No pictures. Keep in mind that now she was no longer objecting to me being present at the birth, so some progress had been made.

Not to worry, I told the nurse, I will talk to Dr. Maugham. Dr. Maugham was notorious for his old-school ways. He was known to stand at the bottom of the steep auditorium at the Royal Victoria Hospital before starting his lecture, waiting for the medical students to achieve what he considered proper decorum. As much as ten minutes would pass, the students anxiously trying to fathom what he was waiting for, when he would say: "Will the student in the top row who is without a tie, please leave so the lecture can begin."

So I went down to his office to explain. "Dr. Klein," he said in his deep and authoritative voice, "we do not want these pictures to be getting around." Getting around! What did he think I was going to do, sell them on street corners? "I know, Dr. Klein," he said, "you think that I am being unfair, but we have standards to maintain. You are being very immature. One day you will thank me for this." Thank him for what? He reminded me of Dean Mary Dolliver at Oberlin. How come all these authoritarians were "doing it for my own good"?

At that point, I had a problem. Bonnie was upstairs approaching the end of her labour, and I was going to miss supporting her, or even the birth itself. Should I continue arguing with someone whose opinion would never change or get back upstairs where I belonged?

So—lovely birth. No pictures.

In retrospect it seemed like Bonnie and I were actually living the slow changes that were underway in what was called in Quebec the humanization of maternity care—elsewhere, family-centred maternity care. This movement in the 1960s and '70s was driven by women marching on hospitals and demanding to reclaim childbirth, welcome partners into the delivery room and avoid unnecessary procedures.

19. A COUNTRY DEEPLY DIVIDED

WHILE WE WERE ENJOYING OUR new lives in Montreal, the Vietnam War dragged on. From 1967 to 1973, the US was a country deeply divided. Champion boxer Muhammad Ali was also drafted in 1967 and refused to fight in a "white man's war." He eloquently placed the war in context when he said that he had nothing against the North Vietnamese. He refused to fight against other people of colour when he had his own fight at home. He famously said: "They never called me nigger." He claimed to be a CO and eventually was deemed to be sincere by a unanimous decision of the US Supreme Court. Amazingly, however, Ali was punished for disloyalty and at the time even considered the most hated man in America, reviled by both Black and white people for renouncing Christianity and refusing to serve in the US Army in an unjust war. His principled position cost him his boxing title and millions of dollars. But at the time of his death in 2016, he was considered a hero for his opposition to the war and steadfast support of Black people in their fight for equality.

The Chicago Democratic Convention of 1968 showed how alienated the youth were from the leaders who pursued the war. I was in good company. People with resources like Muhammad Ali and even myself had the energy and support to win out in the end, while many thousands of poor, mostly men of colour fought and died in Vietnam.

After discharge, physically and mentally damaged vets and the few who somehow managed to complete their service more or less intact were returning to a society that could no longer understand them or appreciate their sacrifice. After the My Lai Massacre in 1968, many considered them "baby killers." While soldiers were away "defending our freedoms" and fighting a war with casualty statistics that could run as high as 80 per cent, American society had become deeply divided about the war. The atrocities the vets had witnessed and sometimes engaged in had turned these young, mostly poor kids into angry and at times sociopathic outsiders who could only speak of their pain to other vets. Those who survived were marked for life, and many returned to the US drug dependent and depressed. A huge number eventually committed suicide.

Soldiers returning from the Vietnam War were regularly greeted by crowds of chanting anti-war demonstrators, accusing the vets of a variety of crimes, even directing their anger at those arriving in wheelchairs. Few remembered that the soldiers in Vietnam were instrumental in helping to end the war, as many simply refused to follow foolish orders that had a high risk of causing their death, without achieving anything of strategic value. Some turned on their officers, even blowing them up in a process called fragging. During 1967–70, with increasing frequency soldiers were being ordered by their officers to patrol an area that they knew was devoid of Viet Cong but full of booby traps and explosive devices. Most soldiers followed these deadly orders, but late in the war, some night patrols would just hole up and smoke dope, rather than expose themselves to useless death and injury.

Though hard to confirm, the estimated numbers for Vietnam War dead are more than 58,200 American soldiers, as many as 2 million Vietnamese civilians on both sides, around 1.1 million North Vietnamese and Viet Cong fighters, and between 200,000 and 250,000 South Vietnamese soldiers.

On January 21, 1977, President Carter provided amnesty for all Vietnam-era draft resisters/dodgers. I never received amnesty, nor would the term "dodger" have applied to me. I was fortunate enough to have been able to create my own personal idiosyncratic amnesty.

It is rarely appreciated that up to twenty thousand young Canadian men joined the US Army to fight in Vietnam. Strangely, given my determination not to serve in Vietnam, and the very different path that I followed, I have connected with a group of these veterans and have been privileged to hear their stories and appreciate how the war forever altered their lives. Many joined the US military for the adventure, or they were just naive. They suffered the same traumas and PTSD as the American veterans of the war. Many still don't sleep, sending me emails in the middle of the night. Alcoholism is an issue. Their marriages are often in shambles. Many have anger management problems. Today, fifty years after the war, many are still suffering. Their organization in Canada is still trying to get the US government to pay for their disabilities.

The returning Canadian vets were often treated with anger and disdain, especially as the Canadian public failed to understand why they joined up in the first place. This kind of anti-homecoming goes a long way to explain why few vets in the US and Canada talk about the war, except safely among those with a shared experience, especially as they know that some of what they were ordered to do was ethically indefensible.

In listening to their stories, I learned that they had a lot of sympathy for those who avoided the war in Vietnam and the Iraq War. But I also learned that they could not tolerate a deserter. You never leave your buddies behind. And here I was, an actual deserter from the very war that had so altered their lives. I guess they accepted me in the end because I listened respectfully to their stories and commiserated with what they went through. Talking with them affected me deeply. Even though I was a physician, I could easily have had a similar life-altering experience. Perhaps my attachment to these Canadian Vietnam War vets reflected some guilt that I had for not sharing their horrible experiences.

In 2006, in the Interior of British Columbia, a reunion took place to honour Vietnam War resisters who came to Canada, and the Canadians who welcomed them during the war and helped them integrate into Canadian life. As part of that event, I was scheduled to co-lead a workshop on PTSD with a Canadian Vietnam vet. Talking with the Canadian vets confirmed, as I had feared, that military doctors were obliged to support the mission by returning soldiers to combat well before they were either physically or psychologically ready. Soldiers coped through heavy alcohol and drug use, the former being very much a part of military culture around the world.

I arrived early for the reunion and was eagerly waiting for my workshop co-leader, Gerry, to arrive. Gerry was in the leadership of the Canadians who had gone south to join up. Increasingly anxious, I called him on my cell.

"Where are you?" I asked. "We are on in three hours."

Talking through his headset, he reassured me: "Don't worry. I am on my motorcycle. I am almost there."

"What's going on?" I said. "Where have you been?"

"Saipan."

"What the hell were you doing in Saipan?"

"Recovering bodies."

"Hey, Gerry," I said, "that's the wrong war." Saipan is in the middle of the Pacific. It was involved in World War II.

Speaking over the roar of his motorcycle, he said: "The air force knew where the planes went down. They just had not yet recovered all of the downed airmen."

I asked him if he recovered any.

"Damn right. Several. We dug them out of their planes, which had been downed in the swamps, and we recovered the remains of the pilots to return to their families. That's what I do."

So there you have it. You never leave your buddies behind.

The workshop went well, though there were moments when the largely anti-war audience would inadvertently say something that would trigger an almost violent response from Gerry. No one who had not had Gerry's experience could have known how reactive he would still be, almost fifty years after his return from combat.

20. MY LIFE AS A PEDIATRIC RESIDENT IN MONTREAL

I WAS GIVEN LOTS OF responsibility at Montreal Children's Hospital, and I thrived. At times, though, I was viewed as a bit strange, partly because of my peculiar status as a deserter but mainly because of my extensive experience at the pediatric hospital in Ethiopia.

DIPHTHERIA PRESENTS

At about 10 p.m. I was on duty in the emergency room. I was very new to Montreal. A child presented in extreme respiratory distress. She was near death. It was obvious to me that the child had diphtheria with a blocked airway. The child also probably had the cardiac failure secondary to cardiomyopathy ("floppy heart") often seen with the disease. The other residents thought I was crazy. "We don't have diphtheria here. We immunize against the disease. The DPT shot does that." The D is for diphtheria; the P for pertussis, or whooping cough; and the T for tetanus. The child required an immediate tracheotomy. But the attending surgical staff was not in the building. I insisted on my diagnosis and asked the nurse to call the ENT (ear, nose and throat) surgeon on call. With the child in my arms, I made for the elevator to the tenth floor, where the operating suites were located.

The bad news is that, as a new staff member, I did not know the layout of the hospital. The bank of elevators that I took was on the wrong side of the operating suites. Instead of entering the front, I entered the back and found myself walking through all the operating rooms, contaminating everything with the lethal diphtheria bacteria as I went.

There was no time to wait for the pediatric surgeon to arrive. The anaesthesiology chief, who happened to be in the hospital, passed an endotracheal tube, and I did the tracheotomy. Together we saved the child's life, in an endeavour that was eerily reminiscent of my experience with Haile Selassie's grandson.

But the surgeons were not happy. All the operating rooms had to be closed for several days while the entire suite was decontaminated. Thus was born a story about that crazy draft dodger guy.

A month or so later, another child presented to the emergency room, this time with severe dehydration resulting from diarrhea and vomiting. The child was in such deep shock that no veins were visible for us to start an intravenous drip to administer fluids. This was a common event in Addis Ababa. We would rapidly warm a bottle of normal saline under hot water in the sink, put a large spinal needle into the abdomen at the umbilicus and rapidly infuse whatever it took to deal with the shock. The peritoneal lining of the abdomen is a huge membrane that rapidly absorbs the fluid and puts it into circulation. This solution was unheard of in Montreal.

It took more than a litre and a half of fluid before the veins finally appeared so that I could do a surgical exposure of the previously collapsed veins. I was then able to insert a catheter into a vein to administer the needed fluids.

LEAD POISONING

In the middle of the night, I was called to the emergency room of Children's to see a two-year-old who was deeply comatose and pale with sluggish pupil responses, indicating severe brain injury. A smear of his anemic blood showed basophilic stippling and many fragmented red blood cells, typical findings in lead poisoning. His mother reported that he had been suffering from abdominal pain, which was treated with clear fluids. My previous experience in the Bronx with lead poisoning among poor children who were eating leaded paint chips had alerted me to the certainty of lead poisoning in this case, but it made no sense. Although anemia and basophilic stippling are certainly the tipoff to lead poisoning, this child came from a white middle-class family from the suburbs. We just did not see lead poisoning in Montreal.

I rapidly began a process of chelation, administering drugs that bind lead, a therapy unknown to the Children's staff, as they did not see lead poisoning. I applied what we did in the Bronx to remove lead from blood and tissue, but before the treatment could take effect, the child died, his brain so swollen that life was unsustainable. While I questioned the distraught mother about possible sources of lead, we managed to get the four-year-old brother into the hospital. He also had suffered from abdominal pain, and the same pediatrician had been recommending clear fluids, with the same unfortunate result. He too was anemic and suffering from lead poisoning, but as he was bigger and older, he was not as sick. But what was the source of the lead?

In a joint sleuthing exercise with the mother, we finally determined the cause. The mother was an excellent amateur potter. She had fashioned a pot that she used to store apple juice in the refrigerator, topping it up when it got low. When the children began to have abdominal pain and cramping, a sign of lead poisoning but of many other things as well, their pediatrician recommended clear fluids. She gave the apple juice from the handcrafted jug that she had herself made, employing the glaze according to the formula recommended in her pottery manual. She had done everything right.

When she brought in the jug for me to examine, it was clear that the pot was lined with a white dusty powder, probably lead oxide. On our analysis, we found the pot released an amazing concentration of lead. Meanwhile, I had successfully chelated the four-year-old, who was recovering.

Knowing nothing about pottery, I joined forces with Rosalie Namer, a well-known local potter, who studied the formula the mother had used from her pottery handbook, which was the book most used by hobbyists across North America. *The formula was wrong.* For lead to remain in the glaze, it required two parts of silica to one part of lead. The written formula was one to one, thereby allowing the lead to be released in the presence of acid solutions, like apple juice.

Abdominal pain from lead poisoning from pottery and pewter occurred often in the 1700s in the colonies of the American Revolution; it was known then as the dry gripes. It was also well known as far back as Greek and Roman times, with cases appearing occasionally to the present. It was thought to account for sterility, and even the fall of the Roman Empire. The theory was that the Roman upper patrician classes were storing wine in glazed pots, whereas the artisan class, who could not afford such luxury, flourished and reproduced.

That could have been the end of the story, but the potter and I needed to know how often this kind of event was occurring. The potter compounded many identical test pots. She applied different glazes according to the existing formulae in the texts of the day and exposed the pots to apple juice. Other faulty formulae were discovered.

I obtained a small grant and gave ten McGill medical students fifty dollars each to go shopping at Christmas time with instructions to buy whatever pottery containers caught their fancy, without telling them what was being studied. They returned with many pots—domestic, imported and handcrafted. Many released large amounts of lead. Earthenware was the most problematic, especially the brown, lightly glazed Mexican pottery that was ubiquitous.

The problem formula and many other incorrect formulae in the hobbyist texts had to be rewritten. With some difficulty, this was accomplished. Rosalie and I moved ahead with the project. The needed publicity was obtained. We then presented our findings to the appropriate authorities on both sides of the Canada-US border. We then worked with the appropriate governmental agencies in the US and Canada to change importation rules to stop the import of improperly glazed vessels and resolve the public health problem. And we worked with the appropriate authorities to develop legislation in the US and Canada to define safe glazes. Our findings were published in the *New England Journal of Medicine*.[3]

Trying to turn this terrible event into something as positive as possible, I spent a lot of time supporting the mother, who was blaming herself. She continued to stay in touch. The four-year-old developed normally. The family went on to adopt a child. I have tried several times since to have research published by the iconic *New England Journal of Medicine* and failed, whereas as a resident I had been successful. That's the way it goes.

PREMATURITY AND THE BATTERED CHILD SYNDROME

I was called to the emergency room to see a very small, very sick infant. It was immediately clear to me he had been severely battered. He was hugely bruised and had multiple fractures. He died of a ruptured stomach. The sad story could have ended there, the parents charged with murder.

The child had been a very small premature infant who was cared for on the newborn service at Children's. He had spent many months in hospital, required weeks on a ventilator, experienced a variety of major crises but survived to be discharged to two young, immature parents. Whose fault was this? Well, everybody's. Young parents are more likely to have a premature infant. And they are least able to care for a high-needs newborn. Teen mothers often get pregnant to have somebody to love and love them in return. This neurologically damaged baby, who had barely survived a variety of conditions and was unwell at discharge, was hardly able to do that. Did they have enough support? Certainly not.

Struggling to process this tragedy, I wondered what the prematurity itself might have had to do with the battering. The incidence of prematurity is about 6 per cent. In a rather simple study, I pulled all the hospital's charts of children who had a diagnosis of battered child syndrome in a twenty-year period. I found that 26 per cent of them had been premature infants. Thus, prematurity clearly predisposed them to battering. And the sicker they were, the more likely they were to become battered. In fact, any child with a chronic disease or disability is more likely to be abused. While I was still a resident, I published the finding.[4]

These examples of my research illustrate that, beginning early in my career, I used a very eclectic approach. I studied what I needed to study. I felt compelled to think beyond the obvious to learn the underlying issues. I could not stop myself. These cases not only demanded diagnosis and resolution but raised questions of a systemic, even societal, nature that required answering. Why were these cases presenting? How could I not try to understand underlying causes? Later, as I began to focus on maternity and newborn care, the same approach characterized my work. Why was maternity care so resistant to change? Why were old and discredited approaches still in practice? Why was it so difficult to appreciate the obvious? What medical care did women really need?

I had completed my senior residency, and because I had been promoted rapidly through the postgraduate educational system, I still needed more total pediatric time to qualify to write the exams that would make me a Canadian and American pediatric specialist. I intended to stay in Canada, so I looked around Montreal to see what to study next. It boiled down to two good choices: Dr. Robert Usher, a well-known neonatologist who later became my mentor and whose work I regarded as seminal, or Dr. Charles Scriver, a world-renowned biochemical geneticist. I decided to do both. The paradox was that I never intended to become either a neonatologist or a biochemical geneticist, but as I had to remain in Montreal, I wanted to make the most of it.

I began with Charles Scriver's lab, spending six months working with patients with inborn genetic metabolic amino acid abnormalities, including phenylketonuria and tyrosinemia. What was interesting for me was not the biochemistry of the diseases but the lives of the families carrying the diseases. Hence, I visited them in their homes, collected specimens and ran the analyses. Although I learned a great deal, including appreciation for Dr. Scriver's holistic approach to his patients, I knew that this was not to be my path.

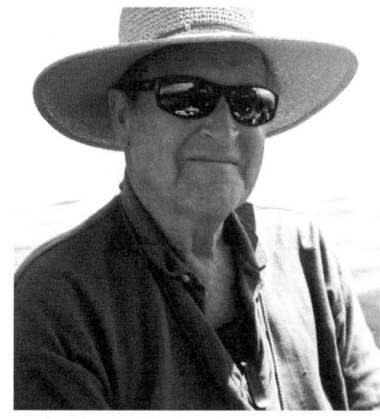

Dr. Robert Usher, a well-known neonatologist and my mentor, enjoying vacation with us.

The next period was as a chief resident with Robert Usher at the newborn intensive care nursery at the Royal Victoria Hospital. I greatly admired Dr. Usher's research and the way he cared intensely about his little patients. But more importantly, I liked him as a person and I liked the way his neonatology unit worked. He gave the nurses great responsibility and engaged them in the research. He knew that I was not heading for neonatology as a career but some variety of community medicine. Nevertheless, I had determined that Dr. Usher had a lot to teach me about research methods as well as clinical care, regardless of where I would eventually wind up.

Dr. Usher appreciated my prior experience in Ethiopia and in the newborn nursery at Stanford. Therefore, unusual for him, he just oriented me for a couple of days and then left for a much-needed summer vacation, leaving me in charge of the neonatal intensive care unit. I was not completely alone, as Dr. Saroj Saigal arrived at about the same time. She was to be Dr. Usher's research fellow, but she had good clinical skills, and we greatly enjoyed each other as colleagues. In practice we shared responsibility for the unit. She later became a well-regarded neonatologist and an expert in the long-term follow-up of very small premature infants.

Dr. Usher was a phone call away, but we tried not to call him. I felt that he was reassured that we would not get into too much trouble, as his head nurses were incredibly experienced and made sure that we stayed on course, and they were generous with their advice. Dr. Usher's genius was in the way he gave his staff responsibility and appreciated them. He was also a wonderful debater, and I enjoyed the banter. I later learned that others thought him too argumentative and opinionated. I never felt that.

Dr. Usher was the father of the early effective treatment for hyaline membrane disease (respiratory distress syndrome) and the care of the very small premature infant. Many other neonatologists denigrated the excellence of his outcomes with comments like: "Nobody can get such good results because he is present on the unit all the time." They called it the Usher Effect, which was a put-down, as in their units, care was passed on to residents and others down the food chain, and the chief was often remote from the shop floor. When we called Dr. Usher, he would even bicycle to the unit in the middle of the night. This was indeed the Usher Effect in action.

He taught me research methodology and critical thinking. For more than six months, I cared for one 615-gram baby, named baby Ho, a premature infant who at the time was among the smallest known survivors at such a low weight. In caring for this newborn, with Dr. Usher's support, I was able to learn what he jokingly referred to as "all of neonatology."

It began with a call for me, as resuscitation officer, to come to the delivery room for the birth of a very small infant. As I arrived, Mrs. Ho delivered the tiny girl. The mother was a new immigrant, and within minutes she said in broken English: "Too small. No good. No want." She quickly got off the delivery table and left the hospital. The baby was both very premature and very malnourished. Over the next six months, this baby had multiple respiratory illnesses and cardiac failure, diabetes, multiple infections and a series of metabolic catastrophes.

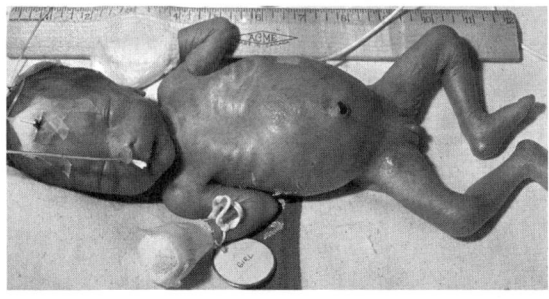

Baby Ho weighed 615 grams at birth. She had multiple system failures as well as repeated infections.

By the end of six months, the baby looked beautiful, but I was convinced that she was deaf, and I was certain that the deafness was caused by the drugs that I had been forced to use to control her heart failure interacting with the drugs that I had to use to control her many infections. The literature showed much later that these drugs, used together, damaged hearing by destroying the eighth cranial nerve.

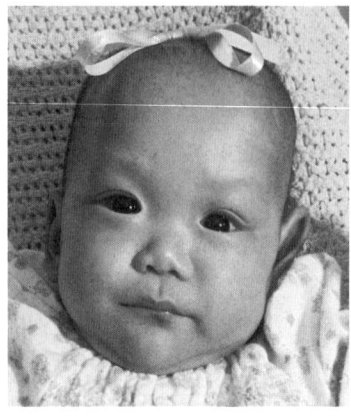

Baby Ho at six months.

Somehow, we kept in touch with Mrs. Ho, who had never visited her baby. But at six months, she finally came to see her baby and said: "Nice baby. I keep." And despite what we think we know about maternal-infant bonding, Mrs. Ho and baby Ho never looked back. Mrs. Ho had to learn English and sign language to be able to communicate with the audiologists and speech therapists. If not for baby Ho's condition, Mrs. Ho might never have left her Chinese-speaking enclave in Montreal and learned to speak English. Baby Ho developed normally and did well in school. She attended a retirement party for Dr. Usher. She was studying to become a physiotherapist.

Baby Ho is a perfect example of the resilience of little babies when they're treated fully for their condition. There was a time in the 1950s and '60s when it was thought that such small babies ought to be left to die. Many of them did not die, but they were severely damaged by the lack of needed treatment. This approach is long gone.

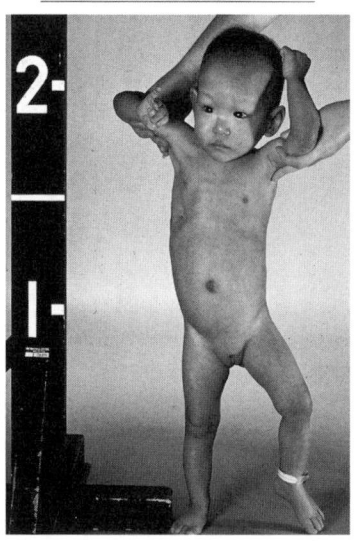

Baby Ho at one year. She was doing well, apart from some spasticity in her left leg.

—◦—

Hard to believe, but rickets seemed to be following me. In Montreal, Mayor Drapeau had declared that adding fluoride to the water and vitamin D to the milk was a "plot" to poison French Canadians. The result: terrible teeth cavities and rickets. The rickets story had been elucidated by Dr. Scriver. It was common in the Montreal long winters to find full-blown rickets, particularly among the poor, very young infants and children of the East End. These children would even appear in the hospital in winter with seizures because of low calcium, an effect of vitamin D deficiency. Under Dr. Scriver's influence, when vitamin D was finally added to the milk, a process initiated decades earlier in the rest of North America, rickets disappeared in Montreal.

After my time with Dr. Usher, I was convinced by the retiring chief of pediatrics, Dr. Alan Ross, who had offered me the senior residency position that I needed to avoid deportation on arrival in Montreal, to become a chief resident at the children's hospital. It was hard to refuse him, but I needed one more year before I took the specialist exams in pediatrics. Taking the chief residency would fulfil that need. Dr. Ross was determined to provide the incoming head of pediatrics, Dr. Mary Ellen Avery, who was arriving from Johns Hopkins, with an experienced chief resident. Dr. Avery was a world-famous neonatologist who had done outstanding fundamental work on the basis of hyaline membrane disease, elucidating the role of surfactant, the material that is synthesized by the developing lungs that is responsible for the lungs staying inflated.

In 1969–70, there were always two chief residents. Normally, they would split the year: six months in-patient and six months' outpatient. My counterpart, Dr. Robert Williams, loved the in-patient and I preferred, at that point, the outpatient. Part of the reason I wanted to remain in the outpatient was that I really did not get on well with Dr. Avery. I enjoyed the community aspects of the outpatient department, but Dr. Avery made clear to me that she felt that the only true science was basic science. She told me that I had great potential as a scientist and that I was wasting my time in the outpatient department.

It actually worked out well, as we two chief residents supported each other and took turns covering the whole hospital on nights and weekends, in-patient as well as outpatient. The outpatient department provided a great opportunity. I was responsible for hundreds of patients per week, as well as teaching the interns and residents. I loved it.

But some tension between Dr. Avery and me developed as a direct consequence of the unfortunate resident strike of 1969. Within days of her arrival in Montreal, all of the Quebec interns and residents went on strike. The basis of the strike was the abysmal way that francophone residents were treated in Quebec teaching hospitals. The English residents at McGill felt that they had to support their francophone colleagues, even though their relationships with their own professors at McGill teaching hospitals were good. Hence, the anglophone residents reluctantly joined the strike.

This resident strike took place just after the strike of the Quebec physicians, a result of their opposition to the introduction of Medicare, which was being implemented when the resident strike took place. I was not at all supportive of the physicians' strike against Medicare and found it hugely hypocritical that the professors were now criticizing residents for their similar action. But for Dr. Avery, a resident strike was incomprehensible. Dr. Avery came from Johns Hopkins, where residents, according to her, were on duty all the time except for an occasional holiday. She felt the Quebec residents, who were asking for duties to be limited to one in three nights, were spoiled. Moreover, she actually demanded that her two chief residents somehow force the children's hospital residents to abandon the strike. "How can you strike against children?" she said.

I tried to explain to her that as chief residents, we had nothing to do with the strike. Chief residents are neither union nor management. It didn't wash. She was adamant that we had the wherewithal to "get her residents back." We felt that we had no power to do this. I felt our role as chief residents was to make sure that nobody died. With that in mind, we organized the attending staff to cover the wards and outpatient department on an emergency basis. We two chief residents organized teaching sessions for the attending staff, who had understandably lost some of the skills that they had not used for years. Pediatricians in office practice do not do procedures or start intravenous drips or engage in the many day-to-day tasks that hospitalized children need.

Although most of the attending staff respected what the residents were doing and realized the necessity, they were not happy, as it interfered with their office and specialist practices and income, so they hoped for a rapid resolution. They were so unhappy that after a few weeks some staff members got a bit threatening. Notable among them was Dr. Leo Stern, head of neonatology at Children's, who somehow felt that I personally not only could but should stop the strike. He actually threatened me: "If you do not stop the strike, I will make sure that you never get a job anywhere in North America." Years later, when I was job hunting, I was told that he was doing just what he promised. But I was also told not to worry, as he was recognized as a bad actor and would be ignored.

21. JOB HUNTING

It was December 26, 1969. After being on duty at Montreal Children's Hospital over Christmas, and now that I was a security risk and/or a homosexual, for the first time since our arrival at Montreal airport in 1967, we were heading south for a family vacation. I was somewhat concerned about how I would be received at the US border. Was there a warrant for my arrest? I knew this was illogical, as I was no longer in the grip of the US government. Soon, I became more worried about the snow, which had been falling for two days and was getting worse. But I was determined to gather our family and catch the flight from New York to Puerto Rico in a few days. We crossed the US border at Plattsburgh, New York, without incident, but the Northway was impassable despite our snow tires, so we holed up in a motel to wait it out.

During the night, a local farmer plowed the motel parking lot, but at 7 a.m. it looked like he had never been there. Snow had built up to the headlights of our little Volkswagen Squareback.

"When's the farmer coming back?" I asked the motel owner.

"You are not going anywhere today," he replied.

Pigheaded me, I began to shovel, first the car and then a path out of the parking lot to the road. We were on our way—almost two-year-old Seth in a car seat in the back and Bonnie, pregnant with Naomi, navigating in the front. Hitting the Northway, we plowed through the first drift of many. I had to get up speed to successfully get through these drifts, but it was unnerving to realize that something might be buried within them.

All day we drove, planning to intersect with the New York State Thruway at Albany. The radio was full of bad news about road closures, and as we approached Albany, we heard that the New York State Thruway was closed. Couldn't be true. I drove on. As we reached Albany, *of course* it was closed because of the massive record snowfall. We later learned that more than three feet of snow had fallen. So we exited the Northway and wound up on an Albany main street in the middle of a major fire. Nothing was moving. Having no choice, I left the main road and plowed my way down a small street, descending into an industrial area, ultimately coming to a complete stop in a couple of feet of snow going uphill the wrong way on a one-way street, in a deserted area full of warehouses. What a way to care for my family.

While I was circling my car, with snow well over the doorsills, bemoaning my stupidity, a tall, huge Black man materialized out of the snow. He too began circling the car and scratching his head, and said: "Man, I like your bumper sticker." The sticker had the ubiquitous peace sign superimposed on an American flag, with the slogan: "End the War in Vietnam—Bring Our Boys Home." Turned out he was one day back from Vietnam.

Concerned for Seth and Bonnie, he led us all into one of the warehouses, which was actually occupied, a home for several families. It was cozy and warm, full of kids playing with their new battery-driven Christmas toys. Bonnie and Seth were warmed and fed, while my good Samaritan insisted on knowing my story. I worried about sharing too much, as I was in fact a deserter, whereas my host and friends were typical draftees. I need not have worried. They were all for what I had done. They too would have avoided the military if they could have.

After a few hours of rest, and with the snow diminishing, our host and I assessed our situation. It turned out that I had snow chains, which he proposed that we apply over the rear wheel snow tires. With about ten of his Black Vietnam veteran friends, he just picked up the back of the car to help put on the chains. Problem: the chains were too small. It hit me that I had used these chains to go over all-season tires when we went skiing in the California mountains during medical school. Of course they were too small to go over snow tires.

Not to be deterred, my host took me into his machine shop and manufactured the needed extra links so that the chains would fit. Again, the car was lifted, and the chains applied. Then a huge group of men pushed me up the hill through a couple feet of snow and onto the main street, which had by then been plowed and the fire extinguished. After waving a grateful thanks, alone on the road, we resumed our trip. In a strange way, I felt like I had been part of the collective actions of the Vietnam vets, who were doing their part to end the war. Yes, that is grandiose, but it felt that way. This crossing of the border was a test so that I now felt safe enough to move to Rochester, New York, for my fellowship.

Now that I had completed my residency at Montreal Children's Hospital, taken all my specialist exams, and been certified as a pediatrician with a subspecialty in neonatology, it was time to get a job. The strange thing was that I had always seen myself, despite my skill in the care of small premature infants, as a community and international medicine specialist, which is where I had been heading prior to the army's interference.

I had put my plans to be a specialist in community pediatrics on hold when Bonnie and I had to flee to Canada. I had never heard of family practice, which had not yet been developed as an academic discipline in Canada and was just starting in the US. Community medicine was also not yet established in Canada. We wanted to remain in Canada, with a rational, national health care system, and we were on the road to Canadian citizenship, but it turned out that I would have to go to the US to study community pediatrics. This discipline was well developed at the University of Rochester under Professor Robert Haggerty. Thus, I took a position as a pediatric community medicine fellow in Rochester, New York. For me, this position was ideal. I had excellent mentoring from people who were committed to the community and who would help me develop the skills needed to study the community while serving it. Notable among the many who taught me community medicine and helped me with my research skills were Evan Charney, Barry Pless and Klaus Roghman.

Unfortunately, when we left Montreal, Bonnie had to give up her excellent position at the National Film Board. Then, to our dismay, she was blacklisted in Rochester for her film about Saul Alinsky, who had organized the Black community against Eastman Kodak, Rochester's largest employer as well as a major donor to the public broadcasting station and university film and television programs. Bonnie survived professionally by starting an independent community video program in inner-city Rochester. Expanding on her NFB Challenge for Change experience, she trained community members to record their own experiences, using heavy "portable" video equipment that is nothing like the light, easy-to-use equipment of today. Bonnie also was fully engaged with our two little children, Seth and Naomi. Despite her very positive activities, Bonnie disliked Rochester, feeling that it was a smug and seriously conservative town run by an old boys' network.

As part of my fellowship, I worked as a pediatrician in an inner-city program called the Rochester Neighborhood Health Center. It ran on a multi-specialty model: pediatricians, internists, psychiatrists, obstetricians and other health care providers all trying to work together with multi-problem inner-city families. I felt that it was a poor model, but I did not know what would be better. It seemed that only the family nurse practitioner had a handle on the whole picture, knowing the entire family. It was unreasonable to expect stressed, often one-parent families to make appointments with each of the specialists. It just did not seem right.

I acquired some further research skills, published a paper on how the neighbourhood health centres in Rochester reduced hospital admissions of inner-city children and did some work on lead poisoning, which was almost as common as in the Bronx, with inner-city children eating paint chips. At the same time, within the fellowship, I was developing a network of neighbourhood health centres on the west side of Rochester. I was both chief executive and medical director. The developing network included one centre in a new Black housing development, one in a largely Puerto Rican and poor white neighbourhood, and one in a mixed-race middle-class neighbourhood. Paradoxically, I had developed these health centres with a US government grant, the very same government that I had been fighting over my resistance to the Vietnam War. Go figure!

While I was immersed in these activities, Dr. Haggerty told me that he needed help in the newborn intensive care unit. I explained that I felt that I could not do this and continue my duties as a member of the department of pediatrics, while developing the health centres. He assured me that if I took on the nursery role, I would have to do nothing else in the department of pediatrics—including no meetings. Given that he had supported me in my neighbourhood centre activities, I could not refuse. So I had a very strange life—developing neighbourhood health centres full time, in addition to heading the newborn ICU for two to three months per year, roles that I continued for five years. I loved the contrast between the newborn ICU and the community. Often, a young student who worked with me in the newborn ICU later took an elective with me in the community and became a community or family physician.

While developing my two roles, I had to figure out what kind of staff would be used in the developing health centres. It was then that I met the messianic Dr. Eugene Farley, a wonderful person and director of Rochester's Highland Family Medicine, a flagship program among the new US academic family medicine programs that had morphed out of the previous general practice programs. In those days, when academic family medicine was just developing, well-regarded general practitioners were enticed out of their practices to head up the fledgling three-year academic family medicine programs. Dr. Farley's program was already recognized as a model for the US.

Academic family medicine developed as a reaction to the difficulties of general practice, which had become discredited because of the limited training of only one year of a rotating internship, as well as negative attitudes among the specialists toward general practice. The old general practice programs were ill equipped to do battle with the ever-stronger, entrenched specialist programs. The development of academic family practice or family medicine resulted regularly in a battle between family practitioners and skeptical specialists who thought that family medicine was non-academic, unnecessary and a threat to their hegemony. In fact, family medicine was a revolutionary response to over-specialization

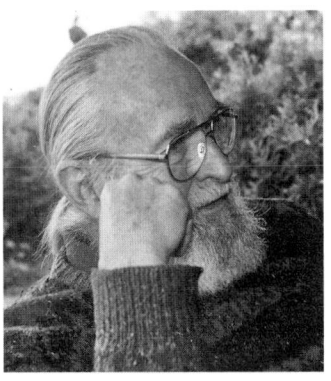

Dr. Eugene Farley in his early nineties, when he was still fighting for the rights of the underserved and for a better society.

and the dehumanization and compartmentalization of modern medicine. You could get most conditions fixed if you were lucky enough to find the right specialist, if you had only one disease and if it happened to be the one that the particular specialist treated—but there was rarely somebody to actually look after you as a human being.

When I was thinking about the medical service model I would adopt for the three developing health centres, I did not yet know anything about family medicine as a solution. All I knew was that I did not want to replicate the multi-specialty group practice model that I had experienced earlier in Rochester. This model could not take into account the complex consequences of poverty and the social determinants of disease. My initiation into family medicine began when, after I tried to meet with a super-busy Dr. Farley, he invited me to come with him to a meeting in Washington, DC. It was an extraordinary meeting, not because of the meeting, which I don't remember, but because of the walks the two of us took.

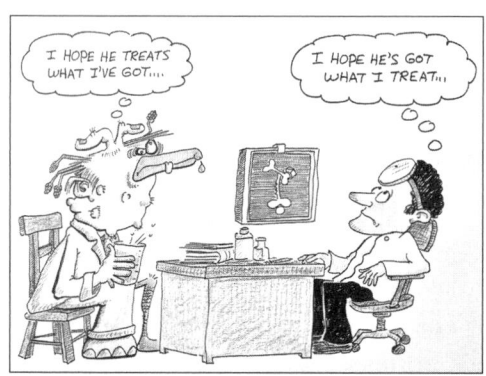

A cartoon one of my Montreal family practice patients, Don Arioli, presented to me after discussions on the state of modern medicine. Image courtesy of Don Arioli

The meeting site was adjacent to "skid row," where we two walked and talked. As we would pass a drug- or alcohol-addicted person slumped in a doorway, Dr. Farley would enthusiastically say: "Hello, how are you?" which I later learned was his usual greeting. We hardly got through one block because he found a need to make human contact with everyone, no matter their station or condition. He was a Quaker, so that might have had something to do with his approach to every human. As we returned to the hotel, he did the same with everyone in the elevator. I was hooked.

Dr. Farley easily convinced me that I ought to run the new centres using family physicians in all three sites. It was going to be more efficient, one doctor rather than many (an internist, pediatrician, psychiatrist, obstetrician) for families that were often chaotic and unable to keep multiple appointments. I followed Farley's advice and mostly hired family physicians who had graduated from his own University of Rochester Highland Family Medicine program. In short order I was able to affiliate our health centres with Farley's program, where we developed a Highland Inner City Division and began training future community-oriented family doctors. Many of our trainees became the first community-based faculty, teaching the next generation of family medicine trainees.

In the health centres, I practised as a pediatrician. It did not fit the very model that I had initiated. Sure, the family doctors consulted with me for pediatric problems because I was easily available, but they could have consulted with an off-site pediatrician. Believing (wrongly) at the time that family physicians could not or would not do full maternity care, the only other specialists that I hired was a group of obstetricians.

As a personal challenge, I began to see adult patients, and I liked that too. It was easy for me to move from being a pediatrician to a family practitioner, as whenever I had a question about an adult patient, I just knocked on the door of the adjacent office, where a family doc was working, and discussed the case. And when I had to admit an adult patient to hospital, I consulted with the chief of internal medicine, or surgery, or obstetrics. In this way, from 1970 to 1975, I created my own unique personal family medicine training program. Then I took the specialty exams in family medicine and passed. I did not stop being a pediatrician; I just added family practice.

THE CORONARY CARE UNIT TRANSFORMED

One evening I received a phone call from one of my recently delivered patients. She was a young Black woman whose blood pressure had been difficult to control. She had delivered a healthy premature infant at thirty-two weeks. Because of the hypertension, the birth had to be induced. Her baby was doing well in the newborn special care unit. The mother was forced to go home without her infant, and she had another two children at home. Over the phone, the mother described severe chest pain that transmitted down her left arm, a classic heart attack underway. I called the ambulance and had her transported to hospital, where it became clear that she had indeed suffered a heart attack, and she was admitted to the coronary intensive care unit.

In a couple of days, she was well enough to ask for her baby. What to do? The baby was on another floor under the care of excellent premature nursery nurses. It occurred to me that there was really no reason for her not to have her baby with her. She was pumping her breasts and was an experienced mother with two other children. I approached the two sets of nurses, one in the coronary care unit and the other in the neonatal special care unit.

The nurses were flexible and interested in the plan, though admittedly it was unusual. The baby was brought to the coronary care unit. The newborn nurses supported the coronary care nurses to help them, or in some cases remind them how to, care for the newborn. The coronary care unit was transformed from a usually glum place, where mostly older men were in bed staring at their cardiac monitors to a place where the crying baby was about life. The coronary patients wanted to see and hold the baby. The coronary care staff assured me that the outcomes for the coronary care patients were improved. Is this family practice or just doing what comes naturally?

22. VANIA CALLS FROM MONTREAL

THE PHONE RANG. IT WAS Vania Jiménez, McGill medical student and dear friend. I was her supervisor at the community clinic we helped establish in East End Montreal, in the pre-Medicare days. Bonnie and Vania birthed their children at a similar time, and we shared values and concerns, including the support of American draft dodgers. Our relationship remained strong despite geographical and national separation.

Vania launched right into it. "That's it. I quit. I will never repeat medicine or kiss the ass of that bastard."

I said, "Slow down. What happened?"

"I was on my last rotation before graduation, internal medicine," Vania said. "I was doing very well and enjoying it. The chief of internal medicine, Dr. Doug Cameron, has flunked me and says I have to repeat internal medicine in order to graduate."

"Why?"

"He says that I have been spending too much time talking to patients."

"Have you neglected anything or failed to complete assignments?" I asked.

"No."

Dr. Cameron was well known for this kind of punitive behaviour. As it happened, I had just heard of a case in the US in which a vindictive professor failed a medical student for trivial reasons. The case went to court and the student was reinstated. I told Vania about the case and we developed a strategy. I reminded her that I had met Dr. Cameron when I was job hunting before going to Rochester. His office was set up so that he sat at his desk on a raised platform, with suppliants below him.

Vania went to the dean of medicine, Dr. Maurice McGregor, and told him the entire story, including her plan to take McGill medical school to court. Fortunately, the dean was a reasonable and fair person who listened, called the chief of medicine into his office in Vania's presence and demanded that he apologize and pass Vania in internal medicine. Given the powerful position of this chief of internal medicine and his history of abusing many others, it was a considerable and unique victory.

Vania graduated and has been practising family medicine for more than thirty years, making contributions in community medicine, maternity care and education. She was named Family Physician of the Year in 1999 by the College of Family Physicians of Canada. She is the author of three powerful novels based on her life as a physician and has seven children.

Dean McGregor's daughter, Margaret, went into family practice and is a well-regarded family physician in Vancouver and a passionate advocate for the underserved, the aged, the chronically ill and the preservation of our public health system. She is also an active member of Canadian Doctors for Medicare.

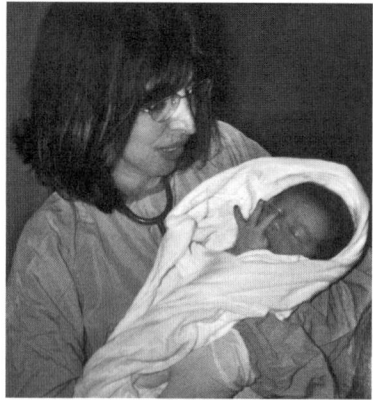

Vania Jiménez holding Elizabeth, her fifth child of seven, in 1983.

23. FAMILY PRACTICE EVOLVES IN ROCHESTER

IT WAS THE 1970S. WE thought we could do anything. Here I was, CEO and medical director of an organization that I had started. I knew nothing about administration, finance, community organization. Never mind. Surrounded by people with a similar "just do it" bent, we somehow managed to get the centres up and running, providing services to communities in need.

Since I had made the decision to use a family medicine model, rather than the multi-specialty group practice model that I had personally experienced and rejected, I thoroughly enjoyed the transition from pediatrician to family physician. Surrounded by the family physicians that I had hired for the three health centres, I continued to strengthen my skills as a family physician.

Family medicine really fit the needs of my patients and was a source of the human drama that I appreciated. I loved the stories. Caring for the entire family provided insights that caring for individuals could not. It was clear to me that I had been destined to be a family physician, and probably would have trained as one from the start, if only I had seen one as a medical student. Role models again.

Because of my large administrative load, I could not have a full-time practice, so I decided that I would only take on whole families. Although this occasionally created problems for individuals who needed privacy from family, perhaps 90 per cent of the practice was truly full *family* practice.

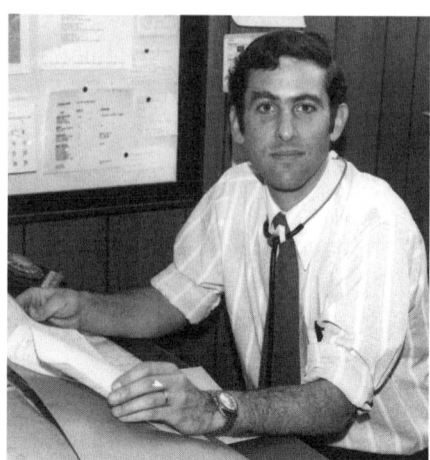

I served as executive and medical director of Westside Health Services from 1970–75.

In the development of the health centres, I worked closely with Dennis Spain, a young graduate of the community dental program at the University of Rochester. A creative dentist, not formally trained in dental surgery, he nevertheless did lots of dental surgery, while also designing and building most of the dental equipment. We were developing our organizational skills along with our clinical practices. It was a bit nuts, and we were bound to make mistakes, as we were untrained for the hurly-burly of complex community issues.

Caring for patients at various financial levels was difficult. At Westside Health Services, we had a good contract with the county Health Department for the care of poor people on Medicaid, with a good reimbursement rate for each visit. People on Medicaid were on welfare, having gotten there by virtue of poverty or even severe illness leading to poverty—still a basic feature of the American health care system. We also had good contracts with Blue Cross Blue Shield for enrolled families working at Kodak, Bausch + Lomb, American Optical, et cetera. This was during the early days of health maintenance organizations (HMOs), now called Managed Care Organizations. But we had another group as well, those we called the marginal poor or sometimes employed. We billed them for their visits and care but rarely got paid.

So we "borrowed" from the county and Blue Cross Blue Shield to try to float the care for the uninsured. Ultimately, it cannot be done and was eventually doomed. Such an impossible task loomed large in my eventual decision to return to Canada, where a single-payer system makes it possible to care for all without reference to their ability to pay. In 2018, the hungry

American multinationals and private facilities are salivating at the potential Canadian market, if only they can gain access under the free trade system.

Caring for so many patients without insurance was problematic. I remember looking into the mouth of a poor Black woman and finding a serious cancer behind her upper molars. I went downstairs to consult with Dennis, who confirmed my diagnosis. She needed major oral surgery and could not pay for it—one of the joys of the American medical system. Dennis implored an oral surgeon he knew to operate for free, which he did, but the woman was left with a huge hole in her pallet so that her speech was embarrassingly nasal. Payment for the needed reconstructive surgery was out of the question. Dennis, ever creative and without surgical experience with such a problem, acted as we both did in those early days: flying by the seat of his pants.

He hit the books, learned about plastics and constructed a false palate, to which he attached some prosthetic teeth. Problem solved. This was the paradigm for much of our work in those early days. I was not trained in administration and he was not trained in oral surgery, which he nevertheless began doing with great success. Dennis later, without a degree in oral surgery, became head of oral surgery in a California facility.

Meanwhile, I began to find the dual role of executive director and medical director burdensome, especially as I was morphing into a family physician in my personally designed family medicine training program, which took considerable time and energy. Bonnie reminded me that this was the time when the feminist revolution was in full swing. It was a time of consciousness-raising groups and experimentation with open marriage. Alone at home with two small kids and a job that could not replace the wonderful NFB, Bonnie joined a discussion group in our graduate student housing complex made up of women with small children and husbands doing graduate work.

We had our marital tensions, largely because of my workaholic focus on the developing health centres. But the dissolution of my early marriage made me determined to save ours. Bonnie recalls that our marriage was the only one of the eight in her consciousness-raising group that survived.

I was determined to reduce my workload. After consulting Dennis, my partner in crime, and with reluctance at leaving the overall leadership of the centres that I had created, I decided to recruit an executive director so that I could focus only on medical issues as medical director, while continuing to hone my family practice skills by seeing family practice patients.

The community board that I had developed and trained was representative of the three communities using the three health centres, with a wonderful mix of ethnicities and races. Board meetings were often charged with local politics, which we were learning about as we went along. Working with the community board, it was a great relief to recruit a personable young new graduate from a business school as executive director. He was Black and comfortable with a good deal of the politics of the neighbourhood health centre movement in the 1970s. Finally, I was no longer expected to attend board meetings, except to report on my role as medical director.

OUR NEIGHBOURHOOD HEALTH CENTRES AT RISK

After two years of the new CEO's reign, Tania, the finance clerk, whom I had known since the early days when I was just developing the network, approached me, concern on her face, asking me to please have a look at several monthly financial statements. I was reluctant, as this was no longer my area of responsibility. She insisted. Even a cursory look made it clear to me that the financial picture was deeply troubling. Unless we did something drastic, the health centres would be insolvent within three months. Tania also had some ideas about where some of the money had gone. I sought confirmation from Dennis, who also looked at the books. On top of the financial discrepancies, there were other personal shenanigans going on between the new leadership and certain board members. As it was no longer my responsibility, I tried very hard to ignore what I knew was going on at that level. What to do? What was our responsibility to the network that we had worked so hard to develop? To be fair, neither Dennis nor I had anything to lose. We each were nearing the end of our employment in Rochester. I had a new job waiting for me in Montreal and he in California. Regardless, we both felt a deep responsibility to protect the health centres and the communities they served.

The operating certificate for the health centre network was held by the New York State Health Department. Only they had the power to fix the situation, if it was even possible to fix it. We decided that the only thing to do was notify the Health Department of what was going on. They would have the power to fire the executive director and the community board, put the network into receivership and take over running the health centres.

We knew that the community board would have to fire us if we contacted the Health Department over their heads, but that was a small price to pay.

So the next morning we called the New York State Health Department and detailed the situation, urging them to come in urgently, take over and save the health centres. Then we notified the board and executive director of our actions and, as expected, were fired on the spot.

While Dennis and I were packing up our things, the New York State board came in rapidly and fired the community board and the executive director, took over our network and saved the health centres. The whole story can be found in the administrative case studies at the Sloan School of Management at MIT in Cambridge. What a way to be famous.

I last visited Rochester in 2009. Two of the three centres were still running and doing well. One of my old patients, who was a nurse, was now the director of one centre. It felt good. At a recent meeting of the North American Primary Care Research Group, I noticed the label *Westside Health Services: Brown Square*, one of the three original centres, on the lapel of a young family physician presenting a paper at the meeting. I introduced myself. "Oh, you're Michael Klein. I'm using some of the health education pamphlets you wrote way back in the 1970s." Did she know anything about the saga of the centres and my firing? No, she did not. Organizational memory is thin.

24. RETURN TO MONTREAL

IN 1975, I WAS RECRUITED back to Montreal to head up the Department of Family Medicine and the Herzl Family Practice Centre, a McGill family medicine teaching unit at the Jewish General Hospital (JGH). We had never wanted to leave Montreal in the first place. If the training programs that I required had existed in Canada in 1970, we would never have left for Rochester. Bonnie was invited to return to the NFB to become part of Studio D, the newly founded women's studio, where she was one of the few experienced women directors. We were ecstatic. Good jobs in a place we really wanted to return to.

But my decision to return to Montreal and McGill was an interesting professional choice. McGill was the last university in Canada to develop a department of family medicine. Montreal was perhaps the most specialist-dominated city in Canada, and although McGill knew that such a department needed to be established, it was done under considerable skepticism and duress. The first university family medicine head was a cardiologist, and specialists headed all the other family medicine units. I was kosher as a retreaded pediatrician.

The position at the Jewish General Hospital covered a large area of responsibility. It involved being responsible for all activities of the more than one hundred family doctors working in the institution, who for the most part worked out of their offices. Most admitted adults to the hospital and looked after them in cooperation with specialists. There was no family practice ward. None attended births, though some had in previous decades. I was also to be director of the Herzl Family Practice Centre, the first of the McGill family practice training sites. I inherited responsibility for training twelve family practice residents per year who would spend two years at the Jewish General Hospital and the Herzl Family Practice Centre, then take the required examination to become specialists in family medicine of the College of Family Physicians of Canada.

The Herzl Family Practice Centre began as a two-bed dispensary on the docks of Montreal in the early 1900s, serving the needs of new Jewish immigrants as they literally came off the boat. The Herzl dispensary reflected the pattern of immigration and the movement of Jews uptown from the docks to the area around Saint Lawrence Boulevard, where Jews established businesses, and later to more upscale neighbourhoods. The original Herzl health centre was also a destination for European Jews fleeing the Nazis. It shared a building on Jeanne-Mance Street with a Hebrew orphanage that received parentless children of the Holocaust.

Visiting the original site, and hearing from Dr. Joe Leavitt, the then ninety-five-year-old former Herzl superintendent, I learned that in the 1940s, "every Jewish kid had their tonsils out on this porcelain table. Saturday mornings was when it happened. Look at my hands. I used to hold the kids while we fluoroscoped them." And indeed his hands showed the degenerative changes you would expect from the exposure to X-rays. He then showed me the key to the front door, which he still carried so many years later. Today you can still see above the door the original lettering in Hebrew, then Italian, then Vietnamese—the history of successive migrations to Montreal.

The Herzl dispensary became the Herzl health centre when it merged with the Jewish General Hospital shortly before I became its director in 1975. You can imagine Jewish doctors in the 1920s fighting discrimination in the Anglo-Saxon, anti-Semitic Montreal hospitals. So they met at the prior Herzl health centre to plan the development of the future Jewish General Hospital, where Jewish doctors would finally be welcome, based on their ability and skills. Prior to the development of the JGH, Jews were unable to gain admission into McGill and other medical schools, and specializing was not possible. If one finally got into medical school, all that was available was a rotating internship as an entranceway to general practice. Paradoxically, the now-specialist Jewish doctors who had been excluded from specialization before there was a Jewish General Hospital, were now making it hard for Jewish general practitioners to practise the very skills that their predecessors employed as GPs in the old days.

My predecessor at Herzl and the Department of Family Medicine was Isaac Tannenbaum. Issie was a marvellous man who was one of the very first of the group of general practitioners who developed the College of Family Physicians of Canada. He was a respected GP who knew that academic family medicine was the way forward. He was the steward who presided over the merger of the Herzl health centre with the Jewish General. Always knowing that he was doing this only to get it going, he was part of the committee that recruited me.

He took me through the complex history and protected me from the sometimes strange personalities of other chiefs and community characters. I will always remember his look of relief as he handed me the reins and said, smiling, "Thank God! Finally, I can return to full-time general practice." Issie was always there for me as an advisor and confidant.

As the new director of the Department of Family Medicine and the Herzl Family Practice Centre, charged with training the next generation of family doctors, I found that I was still dealing with a legacy of discrimination toward general practitioners. I remember being welcomed by the JGH chief of internal medicine: "Now you are finally going to shape up those GPs," he said, seemingly forgetting that I was one of them. Within a few years, GPs in my department were running the emergency room and the neurology and orthopaedic wards (on request of the neurologist and surgeons), and had their own ward where they admitted their patients—and delivering babies would come soon.

Life at Herzl was just what I hoped it would be. As director, I was able to experiment with different ways of delivering services. The populations were extremely varied in their racial and linguistic mix. Although the hospital was the Jewish General, it was located in a neighbourhood where many new immigrants settled. The patients came from every culture and spoke many languages. For me to work well with the French-Canadian population, I built into my first contract a six-month period when I would study French at the Université de Montréal, before I began seeing patients. Before beginning practice, to consolidate my French, I asked my secretary to book only French-Canadian patients for six months.

One of the most satisfying groups to care for was the new immigrants. In the 1970s, fleeing persecution in Morocco, Syria and other Middle Eastern countries, many stressed new Jewish immigrants to Canada flocked to Herzl. Not infrequently, the move had upended the family power structure. In their previous life, the man of the house was usually a business owner. He felt strong and in charge. His wife stayed home and managed the house, usually with servants. Now the man was unemployed and depressed, his skills not in demand. His wife took on the family leadership role, to which she was unaccustomed, causing her great stress.

One day a woman, a new immigrant, presented to my office. In French, she said, "Doctor, I swallowed my tonsils." This is a defined condition with a fancy name: globus hystericus. It is the feeling of choking or being overwhelmed to the extent that it feels like drowning. It is a clear psychosomatic symptom—the psychological expression of an overwhelmed life. It is important to realize that in a family practice, patients usually present with physical or somatic symptoms. If they thought their symptoms were psychological, they probably would take themselves to the office of a psychologist or psychiatrist. In my view, it is important that in treating such patients, you don't make things worse by telling them that it is all in their heads, even though it might be.

My approach in this case was unconventional in the extreme and a bit dicey. I examined her and of course found her tonsils in place. I excused myself and went into the hall to have a think. Then I came up with a bizarre idea. I called my friend, the chief of otolaryngology (ear, nose and throat) to explain the situation. I asked him if he would be willing to put on his head mirror and bring out the longest forceps in his office, then in an exaggerated manner, reach into the patient's mouth and down her throat. In a theatrical manner, he would then assure her that he had retrieved her tonsils. He thought that this was crazy and possible malpractice but reluctantly agreed. The treatment was completely successful. The patient and her family remained patients for many years. Gradually, as they worked through their acclimatization problems, psychosomatic symptoms vanished. This case is perhaps the most extreme example of what we called the immigrant syndrome—always a challenge but very satisfying to treat.

In Quebec, the CLSCs (community health centres) were developed in the 1970s and '80s, after Medicare came to Canada. They are comprehensive units that include doctors, nurses (often including nurse practitioners), social workers and mental health workers, all under one roof. They were designed to meet community needs, initially in areas of high need and later in many other communities, including rural. In some settings, the only medical care available is through the local CLSC. One of the effects of this development was to encourage new family practice graduates not to open private solo practices but to work on salary or sessional (payment by day or half day) payments funded by the government. Herzl was in fact a precursor of the CLSCs, long before Medicare.

When I arrived in Montreal, fee-for-service was the predominant financial model in Canadian health care. Billing for visits or individual acts was a complex and time-consuming activity. This model encourages short, focused visits, as the more patients seen, the greater the income. It is a problematic payment method for difficult or complex patients. Anyone with more than one issue or complaint needs more time. Older patients almost by definition have issues in many parts of their bodies. For such patients, holistic family practice requires at least a half-hour per visit.

A salary or a sessional payment allows the doctor to spend the extra time for folks who need it. A mix of different types of payment methods (fee-for-service or act, sessional and salary) allows the physician to allocate patients who need more time to the right type of payment model. We used this approach at Herzl, with good results. The failure to be able to do this in Rochester had resulted in our inability to afford quality care for those who could not pay for our services. Only by returning to Canada, and a single-payer system, could my personal and political ideals be realized.

But not everyone was happy that Herzl was meeting the needs of the community. One day in the 1980s, a very angry director general of the CLSC down the street arrived at my office in the hospital. Pounding my desk, he demanded that Herzl (which had been in the neighbourhood long before the CLSC) stop seeing patients in our neighbourhood. "That's our job, not yours!" he fumed. Calmly offering him a chair, I asked him to tell me what happened to lead to his visit. Still fuming, he told me that the doctors that he had hired, many of whom were graduates from our two-year family practice residency at Herzl, had quit en masse. Therefore, his CLSC could no longer provide medical services. "Why did this happen?" I asked. He mumbled something about the docs saying, "No security, no independence, too much bureaucracy," though he was not buying any of it.

After deep discussion it became clear, confirmed by the doctors who had resigned, that the doctors felt that they had no say in running the CLSC. They felt isolated from mainstream medicine in Montreal and felt their future was insecure. I offered to help the director resolve the issue. I was indeed concerned that so many of our graduates felt disconnected from a centre that ought to have met their needs and the growing needs of a burgeoning community of new immigrants and poor residents.

It seemed to me that to develop a stable group of doctors for the CLSC, a connection would have to be made with institutions that were solid and secure, that had built-in educational and professional development and other benefits, which were not a normal part of the CLSC. I offered to link the CLSC doctors to Herzl at the Jewish General Hospital and the McGill Department of Family Medicine. Thus, the CLSC doctors gained the security and status they sought.

The CLSC family doctors became part of the extended Herzl Family Medicine Group. They shared call with Herzl doctors and became part of the Herzl maternity coverage group. They soon began teaching McGill medical students and family practice residents in the CLSC, and consequently, received McGill academic appointments.

The situation stabilized, and the director and I became colleagues. I did most of the recruitment of family practitioners for the CLSC, and many other joint activities developed. Herzl was not in competition with the CLSC. There was more than enough work to do in the community for both centres. The CLSC became an important arm of the McGill Department of Family Medicine. One of our faculty, Michael Dworkind, became the first medical director under the new arrangement.

The point of this story is that when family practice reaches its full potential, it remains focused on the needs of the community. In doing so, usually the needs of the practitioners are also met. I recognize that it is essential to recruit the right kind of physician, one who subscribes to the underlying philosophy. To do otherwise is to invite conflict and professional unhappiness, and leads to unhappy patients.

25. TEACHING FAMILY PRACTICE RESIDENTS TO MEET COMMUNITY NEEDS

FOR FAMILY PRACTICE TO REACH its full potential, we needed to select the right kind of residents and provide them with the right kind of faculty and teaching models. We selected the type of family practice resident that we looked forward to teaching. In most ways our selection and teaching methods did not differ from those used throughout North America in the 1970s, as the academic discipline of family medicine was evolving from the one-year rotating internship in general practice, in which the interns just rotated through the traditional disciplines. In Canada, family practice programs are two years, whereas in the US, residents train over three years. Unlike the one-year specialist-dominated rotating internships, family practice programs teach behavioural and communication skills, and bring their residents back to the home unit weekly to follow a panel of patients in the ambulatory setting under family practice supervision. These sessions emphasize that family practice is more than merely being a collection of skills in the traditional medical/surgical disciplines.

Small group learning is key, as is the organization of the learners into small groups headed by a family practice team leader. It is the job of the team leader to monitor the development of the full range of ambulatory office-based skills of the trainee, even when a large part of their time might be spent learning under the supervision of the traditional disciplines, including surgery, pediatrics and psychiatry.

In the 1970s, family medicine was distinguishing itself from the traditional specialities through the publication of the first family medicine textbooks and research studies, which demonstrated that although the diseases that we saw looked superficially like those of internal medicine or pediatrics, the presentation was different. For family medicine, the names of the conditions might be the same—diabetes, hypertension, lung disease—but in family practice, these conditions often presented earlier in the natural history of the disease than was the case for our traditional specialist colleagues. Moreover, our new discipline was developing a vocabulary based on *symptoms* rather than diseases. In family practice, patients often present so early in the disease process that their diseases have not yet become manifest. The central concept is *continuity of care*. The ongoing relationship between doctor and patient allows for non-specific symptoms or complaints to become clarified over time. We accept that, unless the issue is acute and obviously critical, one of the main tools of our discipline is *time*.

For this approach to be safe and satisfying for the trainee, the trainee has to be able to deal with uncertainty. If residents cannot tolerate uncertainty or ambiguity, they are probably unsuited for the work. The joke is that specialists know more and more about less and less, so in the end they know a lot about nothing. Joking aside, for some specialities, it is sufficient to be expert in just a relatively few diagnoses or diseases and their treatments. In contrast, the family physician knows a little about a great many conditions—thousands. It is important for us to know a great deal about those conditions that we see all the time. For the others, we can hit the books or seek specialist help.

The following teaching case shows the importance of being able to withstand ambiguity on the job. John was a conscientious family practice resident in year one of our two-year program at Herzl. When we discussed his cases with him, it became apparent that he was very concerned about missing diagnoses. To compensate for this concern, he was ordering a large number of laboratory tests and often repeating them. He frequently scheduled repeat visits for issues that appeared to have already been resolved or just because he thought he might have missed something. He expressed his concerns to his patients in a number of different ways and inadvertently made them anxious too. Further exploration revealed that he thought often about potential missed diagnoses when he was out of the centre, even missing some sleep as he ruminated about his patients. When the Herzl teaching faculty discussed these issues with the resident, we were unable to uncover a specific or underlying personal issue to explain this pattern. When we discussed his choice of family practice as his career plan, he replied that he chose it because he "liked people."

Our Herzl family practice faculty concluded that this resident was misplaced in family practice. This analysis was not taken lightly. A meeting with the resident, his immediate family practice team leader and me was arranged. We explained to the resident that, in our opinion, he had the making of a fine physician, but our discipline was not meant for him. His intolerance for ambiguity and the reality of never being able to know everything about a case was part of the explanation. We went over his behaviour and the consequences for both the patient and himself. Repeating again how much he loved patients and the teaching centre, he begged us not to abandon him.

I told him that we had no intention of abandoning him. I explained that, in our opinion, he was best suited to internal medicine, and eventually to one of the internal medicine subspecialties like cardiology, nephrology or endocrinology. We explained that in such a subspecialty, he could become an expert in a very focused area of medicine. Most of his patients would come to him on referral from general or family practitioners. For the most part, the diagnosis would already be clear, or establishment of a diagnosis would follow a defined pattern. What would be required of him was a focused diagnostic approach and management that he could master. I realize, however, that some of our specialist colleagues would not be in full accord with this characterization of their disciplines.

I further explained that I had been in communication with the chief of internal medicine, who had made a place for him. "We will transfer you to the internal medicine residency program, and you will get full credit for your training to date. There is nothing to be lost," I explained. The resident was profoundly unhappy and resistant, stating again how much he loved patients. I replied that we need lots of specialists who love patients too. "We are no longer having a discussion. You can accept this, or you will have to leave our program without transfer to internal medicine." And so he went to internal medicine.

I admit that this is an extreme case but an important one. About ten years later, the same resident appeared at my office, unannounced. Rather dramatically, he dropped a package of scientific papers on my desk. "See those papers. I am the author of all of them. When I finished the internal medicine residency, I went on to become a nephrologist [a specialist in kidney diseases]. I have a very successful consulting practice, where"—he said, smiling—"I see patients with only a few different diseases, and I know everything about those diseases. Thanks for kicking me out of your program."

In family practice education, one of the methods used to evaluate and teach communication skills is through use of one-way glass or cameras. This method provides a "window" that allows for exploration of many teaching moments. It is obviously not suitable for teaching much physical diagnosis, but it is useful for understanding human interaction. The patients know that they are in a teaching setting where they will be observed. In fact, we explain that it is not they who are being observed; it is the trainee who is under observation. Patients and trainees quickly adapt to this methodology and usually forget that the observer is there. If the patient feels uncomfortable, it is possible to negotiate a temporary suspension of the method.

One day, while observing a first-year family practice resident, I heard him arguing with an eighty-year-old man about his height, the patient insisting he was a full four inches taller than measured. I called the resident on the intercom and invited him to politely excuse himself so that we could talk face to face. He left his room and came into my teaching room. Rather agitated, he repeated the nature of the dispute. I asked him what it was all about, and again he just repeated the discrepancy. I tried to help him understand the underlying reason for the difference of opinion. Trying to keep a straight face, I explained that the patient used to be five foot eight, but at the age of eighty, he was shrinking. This was normal. I suggested that he re-enter his exam room and apologize to the patient, which he reluctantly did. To make a long story short, the resident left the program on his own and entered an anaesthesia residency. Perhaps he preferred his patients asleep.

26. HERZL DOCTORS EXPAND

From the beginning at Herzl, we epitomized patient-centred care. It was not about what we wanted; it was about what the patients, families and community needed. One of the beauties of family practice is its flexibility. Depending on location and need, family practice can evolve to provide needed services either directly or in association with specialists, nurses and other health workers. At Herzl we were open to caring for many different kinds of patients. One of our staff members began a special clinic for teenagers. Another began a methadone clinic for addicts. We soon began our own family medicine ward where we cared for a variety of patients who did not fit within the purview of traditional specialties.

Some of our members took turns working in the emergency room and a few became emergency medicine specialists. It was all about adaptability. To consolidate family practice as an important discipline, we consciously took on activities that no one else wanted, thereby making family medicine indispensable. This was necessary because some at Jewish General found family medicine interesting but perhaps unnecessary or misplaced in a hospital that aspired to be a tertiary care centre.

The orthopaedic surgeons just wanted to be in the operating room, rather than caring for "little old ladies" who broke their hips. The outcomes of surgery were not ideal, including too many post-operative complications. But with family doctors running the ward, complication rates were much reduced. We were asking and answering the question "How and why did she fall in the first place?" Often, it was because of over-medication. We reduced meds and tried to prevent the next fall. Then the neurologists saw what was going on and asked us to run their ward as well so that they could concentrate on diagnostics and their special skills. Many of their patients with strokes benefitted from our comprehensive approach.

We were also at the forefront in Canada of the development of the formal academic discipline of geriatrics. I was fortunate to be able to recruit Dr. Mark Clarfield to Herzl, who soon developed the long-term ward and established a model of humane, effective geriatric care, and the hospital became a model for the country. Mark went on to be the head of geriatrics for all of Israel and is now chief of geriatrics at Ben-Gurion University of the Negev.

Howard Bergman, one of my McGill student advisees from the Clinique Saint-Jacques days, became the main physician for an East End clinic that evolved from Clinique Saint-Jacques when Medicare came to Canada in 1970. Dr. Bergman's clinic became one of the precursors of the CLSCs. Howard changed careers and joined Mark Clarfield in the development of Canadian geriatrics. He is now chief of academic family medicine at McGill.

Michael Dworkind, one of our first residents, developed the palliative care team at the Jewish General Hospital. He is also a leader in environmental and health peace activities nationally and a powerful voice for reconciliation between the Israelis and Palestinians. Another of our residents, Issie's son, David Tannenbaum, became head of family practice at the University of Toronto. Bob Bluman, David's research partner, joined David and me in one of Herzl's required research projects. Both David and Bob said that they would never do research or administration, but they both did exactly what they said they wouldn't. Bob became one of the heads of continuing medical education at the University of British Columbia. Another of our residents, David's sister Terry, became an expert in community medicine in Montreal. Former resident Maureen Mayhew became an expert in international health in Afghanistan and beyond, and worked with me in refugee health research years later at UBC. This is just a taste of the long list of the work of our Herzl graduates.

Based on the long-established negative attitudes toward general and family practice expressed by their McGill specialist teachers, few McGill medical students were likely to select family practice as their future area of practice. When we selected them as residents in our program at Herzl, they often struggled when our faculty tried to encourage them to plan full-service family practice, including child and woman care. When I came to the Jewish General Hospital, there had not been a delivery by a family physician in fifteen years. To be fair, active exclusion from this area of practice was largely based on pressure from the OB/GYN community in both training and practice. Some obstetricians actively discouraged future family doctors from including maternity care in their practice, and others just made it difficult for aspiring practitioners to obtain the needed consultation. At the time, and this has since changed, maintaining control over the maternity care territory was even apparently a policy at the level of the national organization of obstetricians of Canada.

I had internalized some of these biases myself. Coming back to Montreal from Rochester, where family medicine training was a three-year program, I did not see how in two years, which was the Canadian model, we could produce a family doctor who would deliver babies, when in Rochester so few family doctors attended births after *three years* of training. Hence, at Herzl, as in Rochester, we provided prenatal care but contracted with an obstetrician for the delivery itself. That was my model, but it was wrong and could not be sustained.

27. OXFORD SABBATICAL

AFTER STRUGGLING IN MONTREAL WITH trying to produce in two years a family doctor who could provide all services, including birth, it was time for me to take a sabbatical. I decided to go to Oxford from 1980 to '81, where full maternity care including the delivery was provided based on uniquely cooperative relationships between general/family practitioners and midwives. I wanted to see if and how full maternity care could be safely done.

I was given great freedom in Oxford. I was connected clinically with both the midwifery group and the obstetric group of consultants. Sometimes I worked with the midwives in their clinics, which took place in the offices of the general practitioners, with whom they were affiliated. The GPs provided backup for issues beyond the scope of midwifery, but it was a rare GP who actually attended births. If they attended births, it was as a second attendant, as they believed that the actual birth was better in the hands of the midwives. I also attended a number of midwifery home births in Oxford, acting mostly as an observer, though at times I participated as needed. In that role I dressed in civilian clothing.

On the obstetrical side of my sabbatical experience, I was used as a junior consultant. I took duty in the hospital, attending complicated births at the request of the hospital-based midwives. I dressed in greens with a white lab coat over and wore white wellington boots, as did all the surgeons. The midwives would page me from the on-call room to do a forceps delivery or to be part of a Caesarean section or to discuss induction or augmentation of labour. In these cases, I worked more as a technician, as the midwives had already decided what was needed. Mostly, I just did what the midwives asked. When the midwives called me and I entered the room of the labouring mother, she knew that the whole scene had changed. She was no longer a woman trying to birth her baby; here was a man in wellingtons who was going to intervene, moving her into a more passive role. Her expression would change to either relief or sadness.

Overall, this dual clinical experience could be viewed as a participant observer role. Sometimes I worked with and was seen as part of the midwife team. At other times, in a completely separate role, I was on the obstetrical side of the equation. In this way, I came to appreciate the roles of all the players and how they interconnected.

One of the unique aspects of the Oxford maternity system was that particular GPs and their practices either did or did not do maternity care, especially the birth itself. If they did not attend births, a complex system of hospital-based care was put in place. One group of midwives did the prenatal care, another group of midwives did the care for the birth and yet another did the postpartum care. The obstetrical consultants, in each phase of care, supported the midwives.

In contrast, if the community-based GP practice did provide full maternity care, the midwives associated with the GP practice provided full continuity. They did all three of the components. As part of my Oxford sabbatical, I studied the consequences of these two systems of care. Although some thought of my research as GP versus consultant care, it was really about fragmented care versus full continuity care. In short, full continuity care had better results across a broad series of outcomes.

Because of the Oxford experience, I saw that GP maternity care could be done safely and well in a Montreal context. Based on my own positive experiences working with Ethiopian midwives and with Montreal midwives pre-legalization, when we worked to develop quality regulated midwifery, and because of my former role as a neonatologist, I knew that birth by family doctors could be done safely. As well, I thought that I ought to be able to competently attend births myself. The next step was to develop a safe model of full maternity care for our centre in Montreal. That would wait for my return from sabbatical.

But Oxford provided much more than helping me to develop a model to apply in Montreal. I received research support and mentoring from two key figures. One was Iain Chalmers (later Sir Iain), an obstetrician who was head of the National Perinatal Epidemiology Unit (NPEU) at the Radcliffe Infirmary, a unit doing critical research on all procedures and approaches in maternity care. There I met statistician Diana Elbourne, who worked closely with me on several published studies.[5] Iain and many others on staff taught me more methodology and helped me with my analyses and approach.

Sir Alexander (Alec) Turnbull, head of obstetrics and gynecology at the university department and the John Radcliffe Hospital, also worked with me and facilitated my research. Even as Dr. Turnbull was dying from cancer of the esophagus, he remained involved with my work and helped resolve a very serious academic breach when one of my research assistants stole my data and project, changed her thesis and took all my work and data as her own.

My Oxford sabbatical was partially funded by the Nuffield Trust. As a Nuffield fellow, I was privileged to attend many academic functions. The role opened doors and allowed me access to Green College, one of many Oxford colleges, where I was exposed to the Oxford academic community. Eating at high table with all types of physicians and getting to play squash with some was another benefit.

All the work I did at Oxford became the spring-board for almost all the maternity research I subsequently undertook. Without the Oxford training and support, it is unclear if my research focus on maternity care would even have developed.

One of the high points of my time in Oxford was meeting natural childbirth activist Sheila Kitzinger, who generously engaged me in her activism. Sheila lived near Oxford in the town of Standlake, in a house that was renovated for the second time in 1492, as Columbus was setting out to "discover" America. Her fireplace was so large that you could walk into it. She was a cultural anthropologist whose contributions included a book on childbirth almost every year for at least ten years. These books on education and the power of women to give birth have been used by

Bonnie and me attending a garden party at the Nuffield Institute, where we met the queen mother. She held up the receiving line, as she was so interested in midwifery. She was a patron of the Royal College of Midwives.

millions of pregnant women and birth caregivers. She thought that childbirth had become medicalized and was determined to empower women to contest the medical establishment and push it to provide evidence-based care. She saw midwifery as the central force in the needed changes. She became my teacher in the ways of birth advocacy and changing the maternity care system, a system that exercises pervasive control over women and childbirth to the present.

Sheila was a very tall woman, whose loud and good-humoured voice made her presence felt wherever she was. She believed that pain in labour was real, but women in labour could nevertheless overcome pain by thinking of birth as inherently sexual. In fact, she and others witnessed a number of women having orgasms in the later part of birth. Her talks on the subject encouraged many women to allow themselves to experience orgasm in birth.

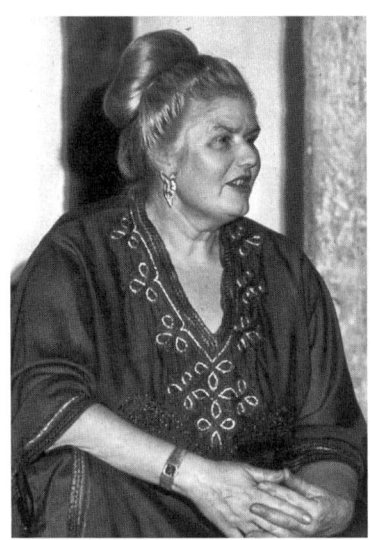

Natural childbirth activist and writer Sheila Kitzinger.

During my sabbatical, Sheila often took me to meetings of the National Childbirth Trust, a birth advocacy group, which she frequently led. To that end, Sheila and I were sitting on the commuter train from Oxford to London, talking as usual about how to improve many aspects of birth. This morning the cars of the train were completely filled with men, with some standing, most in three-piece pinstriped suits, holding their briefcases. They were on their way to the financial heart of London. On this occasion, I cannot remember what triggered her, but she began describing in great and colourful detail, with primal sounds and gesticulations, oblivious to the men around her, orgasm in birth. The men around us moved away. Some began to move to the adjacent car. By the time we got to London, the two of us were alone.

Every time I worked with Sheila, from Oxford to Mexico City, to various cities in North America, it was always a pleasurable experience. Her topics were ever-changing, but she never stopped trying to make birth a positive and growth-enhancing experience. Sheila Kitzinger, a giant in maternity care, died on April 11, 2015. She was an inspiration to generations of women and maternity caregivers. We all miss her and continue to honour her legacy.

I was not the only one who benefitted from the Oxford experience. Because Bonnie was in the middle of making her infamous film *Not a Love Story*, about violent pornography, she had to go back and forth between Oxford and Montreal. I was thus the main parent in Oxford. Seth and Naomi were enrolled in a state-funded Church of England school in North Oxford.

Naomi's experience at the Oxford state school was terrible. It started with a French teacher who told her that he did not want his students exposed to Quebec French, so he exiled her to study hall when he was teaching French. Naomi spoke better French than he did. In the end, after trying to resolve the issue with the headmaster and the threatened French teacher, we pulled her out of the school and enrolled her in an unusual school in a nearby town. It was a town where the European Economic Community (EEC) was working on a hush-hush nuclear project. The EEC was obligated to educate the children of the staff in their own language: French, English, Spanish, German, et cetera. I don't remember exactly how it happened, but Naomi entered the French stream. She loved it.

Seth, in the same state school in North Oxford, had an extraordinary experience. Until then, Seth had been an average student, but in Oxford his English teacher was Philip Pullman, who inspired Seth. It was a major academic breakthrough. We attribute a large part of Seth's subsequent academic success to this teacher, who later became the famous author of *The Golden Compass* and other books.

28. THE HERZL FAMILY PRACTICE MATERNITY GROUP IS BORN

IT WAS GOOD TO BE back home, fresh from the Oxford experience, and sure that we could replicate a similar birth model in Montreal. But the teaching environment was not ideal. Our Herzl graduates, like the older members of the department, were providing office-based care for the neighbourhood and nearby suburbs, but this was a limited form of family practice. Full-spectrum care was the right thing to do. I was also worried that if we continued to produce a family doctor who did not practise full-spectrum care, and who acted mainly as a conduit or feeder for specialist care, the Quebec government wouldn't continue to fund us.

Emboldened by the Oxford experience, I decided to begin the maternity care process at Herzl by starting to attend births myself. Initially, I made an arrangement with our obstetrical consultant, Emily Hamilton, to act as her house officer or assistant when she was on duty and I was available. As chief of the department I had the flexibility to do this. So began a personal refresher tutorial from Emily. It lasted six months, at which point, like a mother bird, she kicked me out of the nest. So I attended births and soon hired two and then three other family doctors who had practised full-spectrum family practice, including birth in rural settings. We also worked with Sally Jorgensen, another supportive obstetrician.

Our family practice birthing group of Cheryl Levitt, François Boucher, Michael Malus, and I were a team. Many in the hospital thought we were nuts but harmless. The chief of obstetrics, in a bizarre twist, thought our maternity work was a kind of feather in his cap. But for the most part the McGill medical students were not interested. Simple office practice, with lots of referrals to specialists, was their plan.

We loved our work, but the four of us and the other Herzl teaching staff were unhappy. Our mostly McGill-educated trainees did not want to learn what we wanted to teach. We recognized early that a happy faculty was the most important factor in a successful program. Without talking to the overall McGill faculty, we began to quietly discriminate against our own McGill graduates when they applied to our family practice program. To fill our program, I crossed Canada to interview potential family practice residents in places where full-spectrum family practice, including births, was the norm. I interviewed medical students from Halifax to Calgary to Vancouver. We enticed trainees from other provinces to join us and, in the most unlikely city setting, prepared them for full, often rural, family practice—including, of course, attending births. I got a kick out of it when one of our residents, the son of the chief of pediatrics at Children's in Montreal, decided to become a rural family doctor.

We four started small but soon developed a reputation for respectful and flexible woman-centred care. The floodgates opened. This influx was in part because of the negative experiences that women had with the conventional obstetrical establishment. Some women had been rejected—in fact, fired—by obstetricians because their requests were thought to be bizarre or unreasonable, or because they questioned the routines in maternity care. For example, some women were fired from their usual obstetrical practice because they pushed back against routine induction of labour based on a presumed due date— requesting instead that induction be reserved for demonstrated need—or because they requested that routine episiotomy not be used.

Another reason they were being fired from an obstetrician's practice was because they dared to inquire about the particular obstetrician's rates of various interventions, or their approach to pregnancy, labour and birth. Typically, they received the answer that the practitioner would do what was necessary and the woman should leave such issues to the practitioner. "Don't worry your pretty little head. Just leave it to me" was an extreme example—leading to the woman's decision to exit the practice immediately. So they came to us.

Receiving this population at Herzl was an opportunity to build our maternity practice and demonstrate our flexibility, to show that we were different from the dominant model of maternity care in Montreal. At first we did not realize what was happening—that the women who entered our maternity practice did so *specifically* to receive what they thought, based on the maternity "grapevine," we would provide. They were very different from women who had been in our family practice for some time and who trusted us implicitly. When women already in our practice became pregnant, it was usual for them to just continue with the already established relationship.

For the new arrivals, however, trust could be difficult to establish. For many, we were often considered as merely the best of a bad lot. Some women came to us via organizations such as the Centre for Alternative Birth or Birth, Renaissance (it works better in French: Naissance, Renaissance).

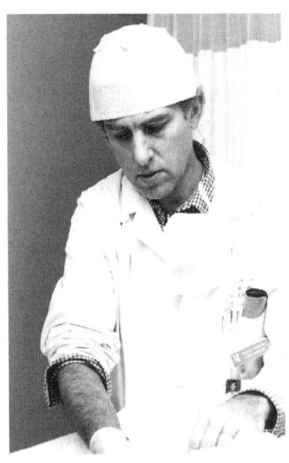

Teaching a Herzl family practice resident how to use forceps. We used to wear masks but gave them up when there was no evidence of their utility in most births.

To demonstrate our commitment to addressing their needs and to show that we all operated with a similar non-interventionist approach, we began meet-the-doctor night, when the four of us would meet every three months with the couples approaching their births. We answered questions and ran a kind of brief evening childbirth preparation session. The parents appreciated that whichever one of us actually attended the birth shared the same philosophy and approach as the others, and that we used technology only if it was really needed. This model eventually spread across the country in many places where family practice maternity services developed and flourished.

Initially, we used soft call, meaning that we were all on duty for all our own patients' births, except for some weekends and vacations. Hard call is when you are on duty only when it is your turn. Before we started our meet-the-doctor nights, most patients expected their own doctor to be at the birth. Although this form of continuity seemed the way to go, it was also a prescription for exhaustion and burnout. In later years, or as we aged, it was common to switch to hard call, even for women family doctors, who initially felt a particular imperative to be at the births of all their patients at all costs.

Unfortunately, our trainees generally couldn't envision the soft call model as a standard for themselves, as they not only saw the exhausted practitioners, but they also worried about integrating maternity care into their future office practice. They thought that this style was incompatible with the structure and demands of a scheduled office practice. Especially as the majority of the new generation of family practitioners were women, the soft call solo model was a big problem for many trainees. They might have said of an excellent family doc: "Isn't she wonderful? I want her for my birth, but I don't want this kind of practice for myself. It's just too demanding."

I described how I coped with patients who had a long list of requests in an article titled "Contracting for Trust in Family Practice Obstetrics" in *Canadian Family Physician.*[6] This was in the era before what came to be known as birth plans. The article was unique in that it was written in about an hour by dictation, while I was lying on my back in a hospital bed recovering from back surgery. It just poured out, which was very different from my usual article that took many weeks or months to write. It illustrates not only my increasing focus on maternity care but also clearly shows the struggle of providing a different kind of maternity care in a city where the care model was specialist-dominated and authoritarian. This became one of my most commonly used articles. Typically, women came with a long list of requirements for their ideal birth. Patiently going through the list was not enough, as the list was seemingly endless. What was really going on was a testing process in which the woman and her partner, who did not yet know me, were using the list to determine if they could trust me. Trust and issues of control were at the heart of the exercise. Although the article describes occasional struggles over control issues, nevertheless, because of the respectful discussions, the patient generally becomes comfortable. When trust and control were directly addressed, the list disappeared.

When trust could not be easily established, I noticed a particular past history. Persons in authority had taken advantage of the vulnerability of the patient, often going back many years, so it is not surprising that the patient would have difficulty trusting any other authority figures.

The most profound injury to the ability to trust is sexual abuse or other injury based on major power imbalance. In my practice, those who could not trust me almost always were survivors of sexual or other abuse. Although they did not leave the practice, in some cases it took many years until the patient could finally begin a truly trusting relationship.

In current practice, so-called unreasonable or inappropriate requests should lead to a written document in which the patient acknowledges that since she is autonomous, she is entitled to make decisions about her care. But the document also should indicate where the professional feels that she is not providing what she considers safe or appropriate care. The professional can thus continue to provide care that may be outside of what they consider to be ideal, or even what the institution prefers. In the early days of our maternity group, unusual requests or patient behaviour often led to the following comment by our obstetrical colleagues: "Oh, another of your crazy patients. Can't you control your practice?" Reply: "These patients have always been there. When you kick them out of your office, they come to me. If you would change *your* behaviour, I would have fewer such patients."

If you delve into an apparently bizarre request, you will often find that it is a test. Unconsciously, the patient thinks: *If I make a truly strange and difficult request, and the doctor agrees, perhaps this authority figure can be trusted after all.* In the end, these "failures" can be opportunities to learn about what is beneath apparent difficulties. I acknowledge that large numbers of such requests can be a major drain on a doctor's energy and personal resources, but they also can be a source of great satisfaction in working through the patient's reasoning.

29. BETHUNE VISITING PROFESSOR

As part of my role as professor of family medicine at McGill, I received an appointment as a McGill Bethune visiting professor to China. Norman Bethune was a Montreal thoracic surgeon who was a maverick throughout his career, contesting many aspects of the establishment. He was a surgeon in Spain during the Spanish Civil War, where he established mobile frontline blood banking. He then joined Mao Zedong's Red Army in the Long March to the north of China against the Chinese nationalists.

Bethune was not new to me. In high school, I had read the book *The Scalpel, the Sword* about his life integrating medicine and politics. In China, Bethune was renowned for being able to do surgery on wounded soldiers almost anywhere. He was famous for training what came to be known as barefoot doctors. Sadly, he died of an overwhelming infection that he acquired through a cut he received while operating without gloves. There were no gloves. Every Chinese child knows the story of Bethune. He is so revered that merely mentioning that I was a Bethune scholar opened many doors and allowed me to learn much as I visited a society that in the late 1980s was just opening to the West.

As part of the visiting professorship, I was to see a variety of maternity facilities and talk about my research on birth and maternity care. It was a strange role, as during this time the one-child policy was in full force. This resulted, especially in the large centres like Beijing, in the false but ingrained belief that Caesarean sections were the best way to obtain the precious only child. Almost all the obstetricians were women. They were clearly competent and on top of obstetrical-gynecological research generally, but they had a blind spot about Caesarean section on maternal request. In the big cities, Caesarean section rates of 50 to 60 per cent were common.

Therefore, although the obstetricians were polite to me, it was clear that my research did not resonate with their reality. Talking about episiotomy when doctors and mothers preferred Caesarean sections is a good example of cultural dissonance. Nevertheless, my Chinese hosts were interested in what was going on in the West, and some fascinating cross-cultural discussions ensued.

There were a few other blind spots outside of maternity care. On the way north from Beijing by train, Bonnie and I found ourselves sharing a compartment with two sophisticated English-speaking Chinese cardiovascular surgeons. They were chain-smoking. We had to regularly escape into the corridor to catch our breath. They were charming and interesting in many ways. After an hour or so of breathing their smoke, and establishing that we were generally open to their ideas, I finally asked them: "How is it that you spend so much of your time repairing the consequences of smoking, when you yourselves smoke?" "What consequences?" they replied. I later learned that the Chinese government was promoting smoking. The taxes on the cigarettes produced huge profits for the state. In 2016, the Chinese government finally launched a public anti-smoking campaign.

Throughout the visit, I was struck by the integration of quality Western medicine with traditional Chinese medicine (TCM). It was apparent that the education of both types of practitioners included a significant amount of crossover, so each type of practitioner was well acquainted with the other, and to a certain extent, each practised some of the skills of the other. At this time, acupuncture and Chinese herbal medicine were just becoming known in the West. Typical in those days was the demonstration of surgical operations without conventional anaesthetics, completely under acupuncture control. Some Western doctors in North America even began taking courses and using acupuncture in their practices. However, in my opinion, based on personal exposure through care for my wife and myself, the short courses in acupuncture for Western physicians compared to many years of training in

China led to Western physicians painting by numbers. They lacked the overall grounding in TCM that allows for nuanced practice.

One of the most interesting experiences of the Bethune trip occurred at Shanghai Children's Hospital. The facility was composed of two completely different buildings connected by a shared atrium. The left buildings were for Western medicine, the right for Chinese medicine. I inquired as to how the patient or family knew which side to go to. "What if they went right when they ought to have gone left?" Reply: "Stupid patient!"

Wait a minute. You mean that it is entirely up to the patient to know what type of care they require? Suppose the child has a serious cancer subject to successful surgery or chemotherapy and they go right to TCM? After further discussion, my host explained that if the parents made a mistake and went right when they really needed care on the left, the practitioners on the traditional side would immediately shift the patient to the left. In fact, since both types of practitioners knew a great deal about the skill set of the other, it was not a problem, and in the best of circumstances, a combination of approaches was provided.

30. BIRTH: WHY DO THIS WORK WHEN IT SOUNDS SO EXHAUSTING?

By THE MID-1980S, OUR BIRTH practice at the Jewish General Hospital had become well established, and our maternity group was active in practice and teaching. Bonnie says that when I came home from a birth, I always looked exhilarated. And I felt that way. A birth is a life-affirming event, no matter how long it takes, no matter if it happens in the middle of the night, no matter how disruptive to my life and practice. It is sometimes a good excuse not to go to an administrative meeting that I did not want to go to in the first place.

Bonnie says that even when the phone call in the middle of the night disrupted *her* sleep, she experienced a contact high. In birth I see women and partners having an existential, often ecstatic or orgasmic experience. They overcome pain and an exhausting event that brings them closer to their partner and caregiver, and transforms them forever. I never cease to be moved by the power of women, and no matter how many births I have attended (about two thousand), I continue to wonder how women manage to get through it.

When I attend a birth, and then a woman's second or third birth, when I meet the children I have delivered and especially when I attend a woman whose own birth I attended, I experience a long-lasting and powerful joy. A most extreme satisfaction occurs when a mother whose birth I attended comes for prenatal care with her pregnant daughter. For a practitioner, attending a joyous birth is an antidote to balance the care of patients with cancer or who are approaching death.

It was time to apply the birth research I had done in Oxford to Montreal. Given my background as a neonatologist/pediatrician and family physician, I often found myself working at the interface of the various disciplines involved in birth. It was logical that one of my first post-Oxford research projects should be about birth.

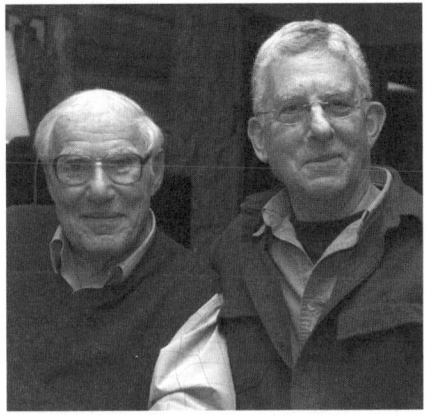

As the hospital was developing its first birth room, I saw an opportunity to study its impact. We decided to do a randomized controlled trial of the new birth room compared to our hospital's traditional or conventional care. To make sure that I was on the right track, I went to Cleveland to consult with Dr. Marshall Klaus, the doctor who I first met as a medical student whose big-picture approach to mother and infant care I was developmentally unprepared to understand at the time.

Dr. Marshall Klaus and me in 2008. He influenced me as a mentor and friend for more than forty years.

As always, I shared my work with my own family. One of the outcomes that I had planned to use involved a newborn neuro-behavioural exam undertaken in the first few minutes of life in the two settings: the birth room versus the conventional setting. One night, as I was sharing the design over dinner, Seth, at age fifteen, said: "The world is on the verge of nuclear destruction, children are starving and you are studying the first few minutes of life? Why don't you study something important?" I dropped that measurement.

Thinking back on this comment, for me it presages Seth's critical thinking and his current role as founding director of the BC office of the Canadian Centre for Policy Alternatives (CCPA-BC) in Vancouver. He has continued in this role for more than twenty years. His thoughtful comment on my research fits well with his current work on climate justice, reducing poverty, establishing a living wage and improving the lives of those at the margins.

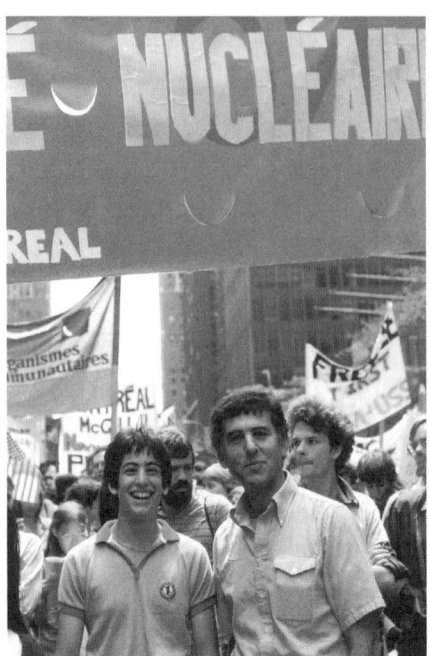

Seth and me marching in an anti-nuclear demonstration in New York in 1982.

We thought that the birth room might have a number of positive results for the mother and newborn. However, the results were at times anomalous. In the birth room, the father tended to fall asleep or read the newspaper in the nice double bed, but if the mother was allocated to the conventional setting, the father was on guard to protect the mother from the perceived dangers of a medicalized setting. The birth room was the preferred setting. Our research showed some benefits for the mother in the birth room, compared to the conventional setting, in the form of some reductions in procedure use. Paradoxically, it appeared that the father in the conventional setting had a more positive relationship with the newborn than in the birth room, and this effect lasted for a year. It seemed that the protective behaviour of the father in the conventional setting fostered a more lasting attachment to the newborn.[7] Then we found that births in the birth room appeared to be associated with fewer admissions to the newborn ICU, a big result that turned out to be wonky. What really happened was that in the conventional setting, if the newborn was not pink and perfect, he was whisked off to the ICU, needed or not. In the birth room, babies in similar transitional or temporary states were handled differently. In that setting caregivers would tend to stimulate and play with the newborn as the transitional state resolved. All newborns did well, regardless of setting. Overall, it was clear that the birth room did indeed change behaviour, but most importantly couples experiencing the birth room were more positive about their experience and would repeat it in a subsequent birth.

31. CARING FOR THE RELIGIOUS JEWISH COMMUNITY OF MONTREAL

ONE DAY A VERY DISTRAUGHT young Orthodox Jewish woman appeared in the office. She had almost continuous vaginal spotting. I examined her and found that she had a small erosion on her cervix. This is a minor problem, easily resolved by cauterizing the areas of the cervix that are bleeding.

Having sexual intercourse is an obligation in that religious group, with women required to have lots of children, sometimes up to ten or twelve children. It is not unusual for women in this community to be having babies well into their forties. But spotting is also a big issue in that community because a religious dictum prevents sexual intercourse during bleeding. Moreover, when bleeding stops, even briefly, the woman has to go to the mikveh (the ritual bathhouse), where she is ritually cleansed and made ready for intercourse. Many times per month, this poor woman was running between home and the mikveh, becoming exhausted and depressed. But I was not permitted to do the needed resolution without permission from the rabbi. What was critical was that it was clear that the bleeding came from the cervix and was not *menstrual* bleeding. The prohibition of intercourse while bleeding pertained only to bleeding from the womb. When I explained this distinction to the woman, she asked me to contact her rabbi to explain her dilemma.

I called. An obviously older man answered in a heavy Eastern European accent that was a bit hard for me to understand. I explained the problem, and the distinction between the blood flowing from the cervix and the menstrual blood flowing from the womb. There was a long pause while he considered the problem. It was news to him, so, surprisingly, he asked me to fax him a picture. I did. The picture showed the location of the bleeding and my plan to resolve it. I received permission to proceed.

A more grateful patient is hard to remember. But that one case led to an avalanche of other patients from the religious Jewish community. When we eventually left Montreal for Vancouver, my colleague and friend Dr. Perle Feldman took over the care of this community. In Vancouver, I applied the same approach to some issues in the Muslim community. Some Muslim women felt uncomfortable having their birth attended by a male doctor. Our birth group was a mix of male and female family doctors. At first we honoured the request for a female birth doctor, but in time this became too hard on the women in our call group—as they needed to be on duty not only when taking their turn but also in a secondary call group for Muslim women's births. What to do? I called the local imam and explained the problem. He authorized his congregation to have male birth attendants when needed.

A STRANGE ROLE

Circumcision is performed among Jewish newborns because of a biblical command to do so. A ritual accompanies it, in which the mohel (ritual circumciser) performs the surgical procedure of removing the foreskin, and there is much rejoicing (not by the baby) and some food, typically sponge cake. In general, I discouraged the procedure, as the evidence shows it is not needed and complications do infrequently arise. It was extremely rare for a circumcision to be needed in an older uncircumcised child or adult because of complications of infection or urinary obstruction. There continues to be a debate about the pros and cons of the procedure, with national pediatric organizations giving contradictory recommendations.

Perhaps two thousand years ago in the desert it was a useful procedure. One can imagine that getting some sand under the foreskin could be a problem. But in modern society, in my opinion, there is no longer any scientific justification for the procedure. The ritual continues because of the history and biblical requirement, and as a way to distinguish being Jewish from other societal and ethnic groups.

The Montreal ritual circumcisers were under the control of the city's chief rabbinical authorities. Thus, although I worked at the Jewish General Hospital, I had no role in doing circumcisions for Jewish families. When non-Jewish couples in my practice insisted on circumcision, or even when other doctors would send their patients to me for the procedure, I would try very hard to change their minds. If I failed to persuade them, I would do the procedure, using the same simple tools as the mohels. My practice was to give the newborn some ritual wine on cotton in a bottle nipple. I kept a bottle of Manischewitz, the official, very sweet sacramental kosher wine in my desk drawer. Then, unlike the mohels, I did a nerve block on the newborn penis. Usually, the baby slept through the procedure, rather than screaming in pain. Doing the procedure without local anaesthesia, in my opinion, is barbaric. News travels fast. I developed an unwanted circumcision practice.

But there was a special group for whom I had a particular affinity: couples who were of mixed religion. Generally, the father was Jewish and the mother was not. Since Jewish identity is matrilineal, the rabbinate refused to allow the mohels to officiate in the procedure for such mixed marriages. For those couples, frantic to find someone to do the procedure, I felt an obligation. But not being a religious Jew, I felt it was inappropriate for me to conduct the religious ceremony that accompanies the procedure. For that reason, I joined forces with my own rabbi, Ron Aigen, who would do the religious part while I was a sympathetic technician. After a while, my rabbi got tired of that role and taught me a minimal ceremony that he assured me was adequate, as he explained that even the father could do it if necessary.

TOO WELL KNOWN

A pregnant Jewish couple entered the practice. They had a ten-year-old girl from a previous marriage. In their previous lives, they were not very religious. They each had experienced a birth in their prior non-religious lives, and in that previous birth, the father was deeply engaged and hands on with the labour, massaging his labouring partner and otherwise supporting her. Things had changed. The father was now also a rabbi and a Hebrew school teacher. They both wanted the intimacy that they had experienced before, but the rules of the very religious group that they had now joined forbade the presence of the father after the wife's water had broken. At that time, she was considered religiously "unclean." I told them I would think of what to do.

A couple of weeks later, the same elderly rabbi who had okayed me to cauterize the cervix of the patient with continuous vaginal spotting was on the line. Without even a hello, he said: "Doctor, how can it be that a woman would need to be touched during labour?" I knew what he was driving at. It could only be a result of the desires of the recent couple.

I told him that touching could be beneficial, shortening labour and even leading to a better labour outcome. There was a very long pause.

"What about the baby?" he inquired

"There could be a better outcome for the baby and the mother," I answered. There was a long pause while he digested the information.

I finally asked, "What are we deciding?"

The rabbi said, "We are deciding that *you* are deciding."

The rabbi had invested me with the religious authority to act on his behalf in this situation. I understood, but given my lack of religious attachment, I felt like a fraud.

On the next visit, the couple inquired if the rabbi had called. Yes, he had called and invested me with the power to make a determination as to the need for touching. In the Jewish religion, the health of the baby trumps everything. Without realizing it, I had said the magic words: "better outcome for the baby."

Several weeks later, the woman went into labour. The father was pacing the hall and reading from the Bible. The woman was beginning to be distressed by the pain. "Is it time yet?" she asked. "It's time," I said. I invited the father to come in to give hands-on support. All went well.

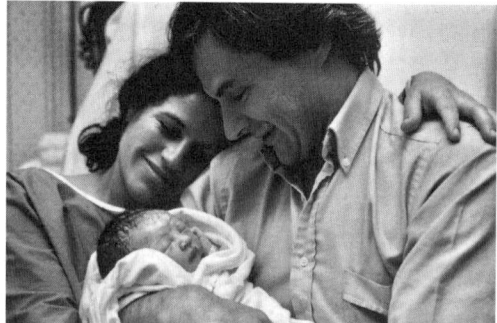

My friend and colleague Bernard Côté with Isobel Orellana and their newborn daughter, Amelia, whose birth I had the pleasure to attend.

32. THE JOYS, DANGERS AND BENEFITS OF FAMILY PRACTICE

ONE OF THE JOYS OF family practice is to care for the entire family. But there are times when it is necessary to split the family, for example in caring for a teenager in conflict with parents. On the whole, the benefits of caring for the entire family provide insights that are not available any other way. Of course, confidentiality between family members is essential. Sharing what you have learned with other family or community members cannot be done without permission.

Case 1: Mr. B. was a high-pressure, very successful businessman in his early forties. He arrived as a new patient, a member of a family that I had known for years. "Dr. Klein, I am too fat and out of shape. I have got to do something about this or I am going to die." He was indeed overweight and out of shape. When I looked in his fundus (the back of the eyeball where the retina resides), I was surprised to see abnormal blood vessels and some deposits of cholesterol. This is unusual in so young a man. His electrocardiogram (EKG) showed a defect in the electrical conduction system of his heart, undoubtedly again because of deposits of cholesterol in the middle of that system.

I explained the issue and the dangers of not acting. He took my advice seriously and worked hard on a medication approach and his diet and exercise. Within six months he had lost a great deal of weight and was in good shape. Rather stunningly, the cholesterol deposits in his eye had almost disappeared, though the conduction system of his heart was still a problem. I congratulated him on his success.

However, he told me in confidence that he was now engaged in an extramarital affair and was very happy. Some weeks later, his wife, also a patient, said: "I liked him better when he was fat."

Case 2: I had a patient with bipolar disorder. When he was in the depressive phase he felt so low that he could hardly work, but he resisted taking antidepressants. When he was in a manic phase he would go to Las Vegas and win many thousands of dollars. He somehow seemed to have the system beat.

His wife and family were also patients. They had to decide if they would encourage him to treat his condition, generally with drugs that would control the chemical imbalance in his brain. After I outlined the pros and cons, the family decided that they liked the money best.

Case 3: It turned out I was the physician for many of the partners in a firm, as well as most of their family members. All of them had stress-related illnesses. Although I could not easily share with the partners my feeling that the business was a toxic environment, I could say so on an individual basis, based on stories from the partners and complaints from their wives.

The partners individually complained of their problems at the business, but they were also complicit in maintaining the toxic competitive office environment. I would have preferred to bring them all together for a serious group therapy talk, but I could not do this because of patient confidentiality. All I could do was counsel them individually about changing the environment. Despite understanding the way the negative office environment affected their individual lives, none of them took my advice. Their symptoms persisted. You win some, you lose some.

Case 4: The Oka Resistance was a dispute that arose in 1990 between a Kanien'kehá:ka (Mohawk) community and a local government over the expansion of a golf course that encroached on Indigenous land and a burial site. The standoff lasted seventy-eight days and led to a sympathetic blockade by the community of Kahnawá:ke of the Mercier Bridge situated between Montreal and the south shore of the Saint Lawrence River. Emotions ran high, with many white Canadians furious.

The community of Kahnawá:ke across the river from Montreal was strongly attached to the Jewish General Hospital, where they birthed most of their babies. Some jokingly described themselves as "the lost tribe of Israel." One of our residents was Louis T. Montour, the first Indigenous doctor in the area and a member of a well-regarded Kanien'kehá:ka family. Dr. Ann Macaulay was the main doctor in the community and a mentor for Louis T. Louis T. and Ann made major contributions to the health of the community through the study of diabetes and the establishment of programs to reduce the scourge of diabetes through partnering with the community in public health efforts. Their work was well known, as they returned the research results to the community, who shared with the doctors in developing public health interventions to moderate the incidence and effects of diabetes.

At the time of the blockade, all of the physicians in the community on the south shore of the Saint Lawrence River were graduates of our Herzl Family Practice Centre. There was an outpatient clinic and a long-term care facility in the community. Complex care and births took place mostly at the JGH. Demonstrating the flexibility and adaptability of family practice, during the blockade of the bridge, the family physicians got to work by boat and helicopter. Some births took place at home or in the upgraded long-term facility. I was delighted with the fine work Ann and our graduates did. The community was their patient, and the patients were seen as part of their community.

33. EPISIOTOMY SURFACES YET AGAIN

GIVEN MY EXPERIENCE WITH ETHIOPIAN midwives, and the consequences during my OB/GYN clerkship at Stanford when I was sent to the county hospital for not doing routine episiotomies, it is not surprising that, as our maternity care practice was developing in Montreal, I might again be questioning the routine use of episiotomy. The conventional idea that routine episiotomy helped both the mother and the baby just made no sense. It seemed to me that routine episiotomy would actually increase trauma to the mother, in part by increasing the likelihood that the surgical cut to the base of the vagina would extend into the rectum. Moreover, although the authoritative wisdom in the usual textbooks claimed that a straight surgical cut was easier to repair, this made no sense. Anyone who has had a paper cut knows this—a more irregular injury heals faster and better than a straight cut. That is not to say that there is never a place for episiotomy, but it is rarely needed.

We four family docs at the Herzl Family Practice Centre did not do routine episiotomy. But I wanted to go deeper into the history of the procedure. I began reading the main obstetric textbooks, from the 1920s to the 1980s. I was astonished to find that in the main textbook, the paragraph on the subject of episiotomy had not changed, word for word, since Dr. Joseph B. DeLee, the father of modern obstetrics, first advocated for the routine use of episiotomy in 1920.[8]

I thought seriously about subjecting episiotomy to formal study, partially inspired by mostly European randomized controlled trials (RCTs) of episiotomy that showed it to be unnecessary. But these RCTs were all midwifery trials and employed a different type of episiotomy than the North American standard. Thus, North American obstetricians could easily reject the results of these trials as irrelevant. I discussed the situation with my mentor and friend Dr. Murray Enkin. Dr. Enkin was an obstetrician and one of the three authors of *A Guide to Effective Care in Pregnancy and Childbirth*, which became the bible on how to conduct evidence-based obstetrical studies.

I first applied for funding to what was then the Medical Research Council of Canada, which rejected the proposal as irrelevant. Their obstetrical consultants could not understand why the procedure merited study, as they believed that all the evidence pointed to the benefit of routine episiotomy. "What's to study? We know the benefits of routine episiotomy," was the response of one reviewer. This was my first experience with how conventional wisdom can undercut any studies that contest the status quo.

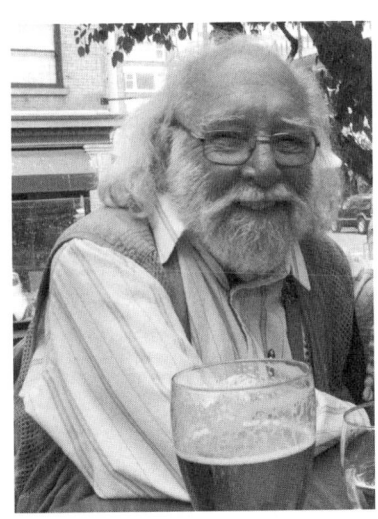

Dr. Murray Enkin, long-time mentor and friend, at age ninety-two in 2015.

Thus began a long saga of seeking funding, researching and publishing findings within an establishment that was determined to prevent change. Our proposed RCT was classic in its structure. It involved three hospitals in Montreal and had a unique feature—the measurement of pelvic floor functioning by electromyographic perineometry (kegelometry). This resulted in a permanent record of the strength and pattern of pelvic muscle contraction, sort of like an electrocardiogram. No other trial had included this measurement, which added an objective scientific aspect that allowed us to see how episiotomy affected the pelvic floor and perineum. By including this measurement, I knew that, if successful, the results could not be ignored.

I applied to Health Canada for funding. While I was waiting to hear, life upstaged science.

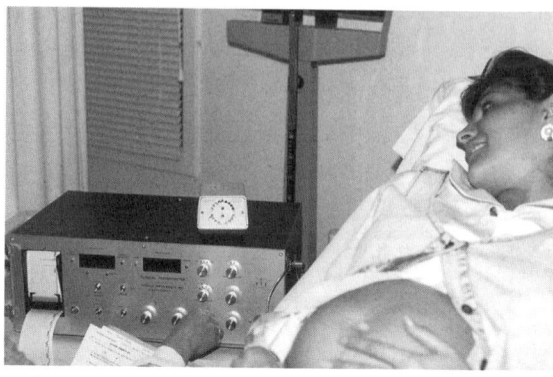

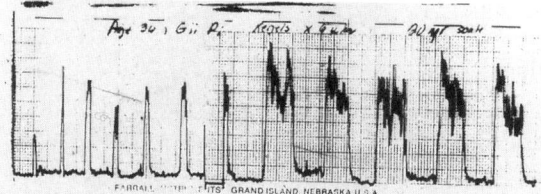

Top left: A pregnant patient in the episiotomy trial getting a pelvic floor measurement called electromyographic perineometry (kegelomentry).

Bottom left: This is what a perineometry record looks like. The woman flexes her pelvic muscles for a brief period and then a series of ten-second holds. Comparison is made with norms for pregnant women.

34. BONNIE'S ILLNESS

On a relaxed and athletic summer vacation in Vermont in 1987, Bonnie suddenly had a drooping eyelid, nausea and double vision and began repeatedly choking. I was terrified. These were brain stem signs, indicating that the insult to Bonnie's brain was near the respiratory centre. While I considered a variety of other reasons to explain her symptoms, I also thought it might be an evolving brain stem stroke; hence, she might stop breathing at any time. I managed to get her into the car and drove like hell across the border to Montreal in forty minutes, a trip that would usually take ninety minutes.

It turned out that Bonnie had suffered a series of strokes, but before the definitive diagnosis, there was much dithering about the cause. Each consulting specialist gave her a diagnosis based on their particular discipline—from multiple sclerosis to a severe rheumatologic disease to cancer of the spine. After two weeks in the ICU, her condition worsened severely. She became quadriplegic and unable to breathe on her own.

Late one night, after I had spent almost all my time with Bonnie, I was too tired to function. As Bonnie steadily deteriorated, I was thoroughly exhausted, sleepless and so demoralized that I was useless. For the first time in days, I went home to sleep for a few hours.

My bedroom phone rang. It was Mark Essak, one of my own family practice residents on the internal medicine service, who had been working alone to cover several wards. He came to the neurology ICU, examined Bonnie and called me. Speaking calmly, he explained that Bonnie was exhibiting decorticate posturing, when the patient shows a rigid posture of flexed arms, clenched fists and extended legs—a very bad neurological sign. I was stunned and dispirited.

Mark told me what he was doing for her and assured me that he was mobilizing the needed physician staff. I thanked him and immediately fell back to sleep. I was useless. I could not move or think.

Next morning the situation was under control, as much as it could be under these terrible circumstances. Pushing the attending staff at the Jewish General Hospital, who thought I was over-involved and a bit nuts, I pressed them to arrange an MRI. In those days, obtaining an MRI was difficult, and it was only available at the Montreal Neurological Institute. We were about to leave the Jewish General in the transport ambulance to get the MRI. The transport ambulance contained two technicians up front and a respiratory technician in back with Bonnie and me. Bonnie required intermittent ventilation by bag. I don't know what possessed me, but I asked the ambulance attendants what would happen if the suction machine failed. This was important, as Bonnie had heavy secretions that needed to be cleared from her tracheotomy tube to ensure her airway was clear. The response was "It never fails."

A firm believer in Murphy's Law—if anything can go wrong, it will—I asked the team to wait a few minutes while I went up to the maternity ward on the fifth floor to get a few disposable DeLee suction traps. This device has a little suction tube attached to a trap to collect secretions; at the other end is another suction tube that the operator puts in his mouth to create the suction. For many decades we used them at birth to suction out the secretions of the newborn. Of course, the suction machine failed, and I sucked on the DeLee suction traps along the way between the two facilities. Note that the suction traps bore the name of the physician who popularized routine episiotomy. DeLee's influence was huge, sometimes positive, and sometimes not so much.

After the transport was completed, for reasons that I will never fathom, the respiratory technician returned to the Jewish General with the transport ambulance. I was left alone with the MRI technician, with me by necessity intermittently bagging Bonnie by hand. The technician did his best to obtain a good MRI study but finally told me that he had to abandon the procedure because Bonnie was moving too much. Desperate, I implored him to carry on. The two of us were alone in the MRI chamber. He agreed that I would hold Bonnie still, bagging as necessary, while he crawled into the MRI tube to immobilize Bonnie from the other end. After about a half hour, the technician was so stiff that it took a minute or so until he could even stand. He was so pleased that he had succeeded in obtaining useful MRI images that he hugged me, while I expressed my profound gratitude.

Then it got crazier still. While I waited for a new respiratory technician to finally arrive to care for Bonnie during the ambulance transport back to the Jewish General, there was nobody around to read the MRI. Numb, I was sitting alone, looking at the MRI film. What did I know about reading MRIs? Nevertheless, I could not resist studying the film. Even to me, an amateur, the defect was clear. It showed a large, seemingly vascular malformation in the area of the brain stem—I thought, the medulla oblongata. It was under the cerebellum. It looked contained and had a sort of capsule around it. More than that I was not equipped to say.

Back at the Jewish General, Bonnie was quadriplegic and minimally responsive. As her condition worsened yet again, I found myself alone over a weekend, with the ward neurologists signed out to a covering neurologist from a nearby hospital who was supposed to see Bonnie but never did.

The MRI indeed showed a large vascular malformation that the Montreal Neurological Institute considered to be inoperable. They offered some radiotherapy that clearly would have been ineffective, as Bonnie had already sustained two strokes in the brain stem. If she continued to bleed, she would die.

Desperate, I sent her MRI films to two former Stanford medical school classmates who had become neurologists. Peter Engel, head of the seizure service at UCLA, brought the MRIs to an international meeting of neurologists and neurosurgeons in Barcelona. He put the film up on a view box and asked, "What the hell do we do with this?" There was agreement that this was a benign nest of abnormal vessels in the brain stem, but in a very bad place. All agreed that she ought to be sent rapidly to Dr. Skip Peerless in London, Ontario. He had been practising on dogs and waiting for a patient. Most such patients die a respiratory death before they get to the neurosurgeon, so neurosurgeons have little experience dealing with the problem. This is because the vascular abnormality present from birth has ruptured adjacent to the respiratory centre. The congenital abnormality is referred to as a ticking time bomb or a bomb in the brain. The thin-walled vessels finally degenerate with time, leaving most patients dead or catastrophically disabled.

At public expense, Bonnie was flown to London on a Quebec special air ambulance while on a respirator. In London, a repeat MRI was done with the help of a special respirator made entirely of plastic, as metal cannot be present during an MRI. This plastic respirator was developed by an anaesthesiologist, Dr. Adrian Gelb, who became deeply involved with Bonnie's care. All agreed that the surgery was extremely risky but possible.

It was Friday before the Labour Day long weekend. Most of the medical and nursing staff had planned holidays for the weekend. I was sitting with Dr. Peerless, Dr. Gelb, the chief neurosurgical resident and our seventeen-year-old Naomi.

Dr. Peerless said, "We will be short staffed over the long weekend, not a good time for risky surgery and the needed post-operative care. We will do the surgery on Tuesday."

Naomi responded, "My mother has had two or more strokes. She is at the edge of death. By Tuesday she could have another and be dead." Even then, Naomi's words presaged her way of thinking. She has since become a well-known writer and social activist, whose book about the links between climate change and capitalism, *This Changes Everything*, and her critique of the way we are handling the behaviour of President Trump, *No Is Not Enough*, are having a profound impact on the climate change debate and discussions on democracy worldwide.

One after another, first the chief neurosurgical resident, then Dr. Gelb and finally Dr. Peerless said they would give up their weekend. The specialized nursing staff were called in too, and the procedure was done that evening.

Meanwhile, I had called a London family physician friend, Michael Brennan, to apprise him of the situation. "You will come to live with me," he said in his typically definitive way. And so I did. And Dr. Brennan and his wife, Dr. Linda Spano, looked after me. They soon had a houseful of all the members of my family, and Bonnie's too.

35. THE EPISIOTOMY TRIAL

AFTER THE SURGERY, BONNIE WAS still quadriplegic, on a respirator and locked in, meaning she could only communicate with eye blinks. We did not know if she would recover, or, if she did, what deficits she would have.

The phone rang at the Brennans'. It was Health Canada. I had forgotten that I had even applied for funding for a study of episiotomy.

"Why have you not responded to the reviewers?" challenged the administrator. I explained the circumstances. I was no longer even interested in doing the study. In fact, I explained, there was no way that I could convince the reviewers of the benefits of the study. These reviewers were overwhelmingly negative, expressing bizarre and misogynist views. The Health Canada staff member repeated: "Answer the reviewers."

Finally, it dawned on me. Health Canada was prepared to dismiss the reviewers' inappropriate assessments and fund the study. So I had a great time addressing the reviewers' comments, letting it all hang out and telling them exactly what I thought of their reviews. It was deeply therapeutic for me at a time when I was preoccupied with Bonnie's health. Health Canada gave me everything I asked for. In retrospect, I should have asked for more money. I managed to finish the study only because of the financial help from the McGill dean of medicine Dr. Richard Cruess, who felt the study was so important that he dipped into his private dean's fund to support it.

Although I had been funded to carry out the trial, because of Bonnie's illness, I was too distracted to actually conduct the trial for about a year after her strokes. The trial involved three Montreal hospitals and showed that episiotomy caused the very trauma it was supposed to be preventing, and that even spontaneous tears are less painful and heal better than episiotomy. The trial is credited with contributing to a dramatic drop in routine use of episiotomy worldwide. Before our study, episiotomy rates in Canada and the US were about 65 per cent, and severe tearing to the perineum was approximately 4.5 per cent. After the trial, episiotomy rates fell as low as 12 per cent, and severe tearing dropped to 1.5 per cent.

Before the main publications were available to practitioners, we began to notice that some physicians who participated in the trial seemed to have been unable to follow the study protocol. They did an episiotomy regardless of whether the protocol card told them to or not; in a randomized controlled trial, you would expect an episiotomy would be done approximately half the time. These same participants seemed to be responsible for most of the severe trauma. In contrast, other physicians seemed able to follow the protocol and avoid severe trauma and have the fewest complications. Because of this observation, as a final part of our study, we had all the physicians in the trial answer a questionnaire asking them for their attitudes about a range of birth issues. We learned that those participants who had the worst outcomes in the trial thought the most negatively about birth itself. They had trouble seeing the women or their perineum as normal enough to be randomized—and they seemed to see the birth through fetal-distress-coloured glasses. They saw fetal distress frequently, whereas those physicians with the least trauma in their births saw birth as normal and rarely diagnosed fetal distress.

With the episiotomy studies winding down, my research colleague Janusz Kaczorowski and I began thinking about the role of attitudes and beliefs of all kinds of maternity caregivers and outcomes. Janusz, a sociologist by training, knew nothing about birth at the start. By the end of the study, his knowledge of birth was monumental. Like those who thought the world was flat and the sun revolved around the earth, believers in routine episiotomy considered its use to be based on "normal science." Obstetricians fully accepted routine episiotomy as normal, even essential. The OB/GYN community saw birth as inherently abnormal; therefore, acceptable scientific questions were grounded in this reality as the only framework for legitimate inquiry.

I found Thomas Kuhn's *The Structure of Scientific Revolutions* helpful in my understanding of the conflict between old and new ideas about episiotomy.[9] Kuhn defined "revolutionary science" as the study of anomalies, or the failure of the accepted paradigm to explain or take into account observed phenomena. In the 1970s and '80s, beliefs about childbirth were coming under intense scrutiny. Worldwide, many people had come to believe that routine episiotomy did not make sense and was anomalous and in need of formal study. In the early 1980s, as I struggled to get the episiotomy trial published because the dominant culture wanted the results buried, I thought about how strongly held beliefs came about and the critical importance of timing. I found it helpful to consider my struggle in the context of paradigms and "paradigm shift," the term coined by Kuhn.

To fully understand the genesis of routine episiotomy, I had been reading the seminal work of Dr. Joseph B. DeLee. I was struck by the way that he put together the need for a new way of protecting the mother and the fetus with the need of his evolving professional discipline. Dr. DeLee was in the process of transforming the field of gynecology into a new discipline to be called obstetrics and gynecology, while wrestling birth away from "incompetent general practitioners and midwives," and he was inventing routine episiotomy as a vehicle for achieving both.[10]

Dr. DeLee's presidential address to what was then the American Gynecological Society in Chicago in 1920 was a masterpiece that proposed a new way to save babies and the perineum and pelvic floor, with his combination of outlet forceps and episiotomy.[11] Dr. DeLee exhorted his audience to take up this new approach, claiming that since GPs and midwives would not have the tools nor the inclination to use a surgical technique, the new discipline of OB/GYN would gain hegemony. His timing was impeccable. Mothers and babies were indeed in trouble in the 1920s—especially in the slums of Chicago, where DeLee had founded the Chicago Lying-In Hospital. Society needed a new way of looking at birth, and gynecologists needed a strengthened discipline. To accomplish this, they had to situate themselves as scientifically providing the solution to a problem. Under DeLee's influence, gynecologists created a new way of viewing birth—changing it from a natural phenomenon to a process fraught with danger, a danger that would be mitigated by the new discipline of obstetrics and gynecology. And society was ready for this way of seeing birth. Thomas Kuhn would say that the old paradigm was about to be shifted.

Having struggled for funding, now I struggled to publish results that contested conventional wisdom. Now the peer reviewers for the journals that I submitted to made misogynistic comments and were harsh in their desire to see the research disappear. I wrote about this fascinating process, using the reviewers' actual words as the raw material.[12] I appreciated that the reviewers were in a different place from our research group. I was not angry at their responses. It was all grist for the mill. What do you expect when you are fighting the current paradigm?

It was unusual for a researcher/author to call a journal editor to complain, but that is what I did. I read to him some of the reviewers' comments. Editors want their journal to be cutting edge and often controversial. He sent the paper out to a new, carefully selected group of reviewers. The journal then published a series of our episiotomy papers.[13] Our results not only showed that episiotomy caused the most severe form of trauma but was more painful than spontaneous tears, interfered with resumption of sexual intercourse and had negative effects on the pelvic floor.[14] When the research was finally published, it was because the discipline of OB/GYN had within its leadership a key editor, who was also skeptical of the old orthodoxy and believed that routine episiotomy should be studied.

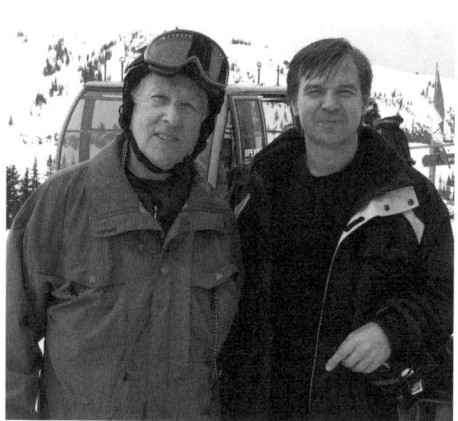

My colleague Janusz Kaczorowski (right) and me taking a break from research.

Janusz and I found that belief structures about episiotomy were firmly grounded in a strongly held paradigm of birth. If you knew how practitioners saw episiotomy, you knew how they viewed birth itself. Our timing was perfect, in line with a rapidly evolving scientific revolution, with obstetrics and gynecology reluctantly becoming evidence-based across a whole range of procedures in common use.

Today, there remain only a few holdouts who still believe that routine episiotomy is beneficial and deny the improvements in perineal and pelvic floor health that accrued from abandonment of routine episiotomy. The new generation of practitioners accepts that routine episiotomy causes the very trauma that it was supposed to prevent.

They use it judiciously, which has resulted in a dramatic reduction in its use in North America and a parallel reduction in severe trauma. Those who still cling to the regular use of episiotomy will retire. We can only hope that evidence of the problems with overuse of Caesarean section will follow a similar course, but it is going to be difficult.

It is rare for family doctors to lead the way in obstetrical care or to successfully contest conventional practice, as obstetricians are considered the experts. But since our group led the way on the episiotomy story in our Montreal hospital setting, it was an easy step for us to engage in other ways. As our family practice maternity group expanded, I became aware of the use of soft cup vacuum extraction as a possible replacement, in some clinical situations, for the more invasive and potentially dangerous metal forceps. The disposable single-use device is like a mini toilet plunger, which is placed on the scalp of a fetus and attached to a handheld low intensity suction pump for the purpose of assisting the mother to birth her baby in the final stages of labour. The soft plastic cup is more forgiving than metal forceps, in that it just magnifies the mother's own efforts at delivering her baby. The use of forceps requires more skill than vacuum, so vacuum is very useful for family doctors, as few family doctors feel comfortable using forceps. As well, it is often unnecessary to do an episiotomy with the device. Typically, the vacuum is applied when the fetal head is low on the pelvic floor, or when the fetal head is almost crowning, but the woman is still unable to complete the birth. In the ideal situation, as the fetal head approaches full crowning, the cup is removed and the birth proceeds without the vacuum—and the mother feels, as she should, that she birthed her baby herself. I always prepared the mother by emphasizing that it was her birth experience, and that we would use the vacuum together.

When I became aware of the benefits of the device, I tried to interest the hospital OB/GYN department in obtaining some of the devices, but they were not interested. Real men use metal. So I bought some of the devices and pumps. The manufacturer supplies the plastic cups and attached handles in sterile plastic bags, some of which I stored in my locker in the maternity suite. When I began to use the vacuums, the nurses were at first skeptical but soon supportive, as they saw that problems were being solved in a less invasive and potentially dangerous way. I began to make myself available to other family doctors to assist if requested. Soon, some of the OB residents were intrigued and asked me to teach them. In a short time, the OB/GYN department purchased the devices and made them available as a part of normal practice.

Compared to the struggle around the limitation of episiotomy to specific indications, this little episode about changing practice seemed unusually easy to implement. Perhaps it was because, in the end, it did not challenge the conventional power structure. Forceps still had a place in obstetrical practice, and vacuum was still a tool that normally would not be used by midwives. Dr. DeLee would probably have approved. While we were making this change locally, in many other hospitals, family doctors and obstetricians were embracing the use of vacuum as a substitute for forceps for some indications. In fact, obstetricians were restricting their own use of forceps, especially high and rotational forceps, preferring Caesarean section as a solution for most complex arrests of labour, which has resulted in the loss of an important skill set and contributed to the rising Caesarean section rate.

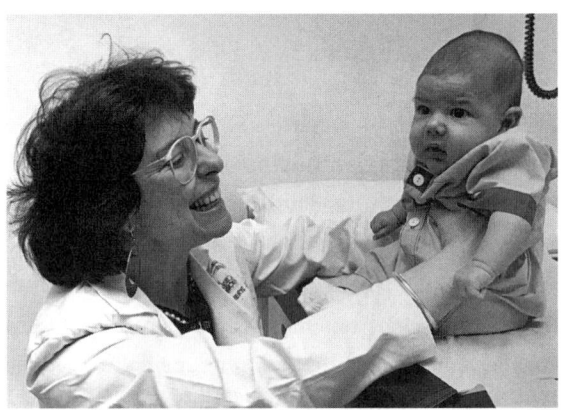

Dr. Cheryl Levitt and baby. Cheryl replaced me during Bonnie's illness and later became chief of family practice when we left for Vancouver. Later she became academic head of family practice at McMaster University.

36. BONNIE BEATS THE ODDS

ALTHOUGH CONVENTIONAL WISDOM HOLDS THAT stroke recovery reaches its final state by six months, Bonnie continued to improve over fifteen or more years. She had a permanently paralyzed vocal cord and was told she would never talk again. She talks perfectly. She walks a few steps with canes and uses a walker indoors, but because she has severe balance problems she uses an electric scooter outside. She is virtually independent, taking public transportation with her scooter and at times with her assistance dog, Luna. We are able to bicycle together, with her riding a low-slung electric-assisted tricycle. Bonnie has become an advocate for people living with all kinds of disabilities and has done radio programs and written articles. She wrote a book called *Slow Dance: A Story of Stroke, Love and Disability* that details her recovery and struggle to be independent.[15] It is a resource frequently used by stroke survivors, available on Amazon and in libraries. Much later, she made the film *Shameless: The Art of Disability* for the NFB.[16] Nine years after Bonnie's stroke, I wrote a companion piece, "Too Close for Comfort?" for the January 1997 *Canadian Medical Association Journal*, which describes the complex role of physician-husband, advocating and sometimes interfering with the care of close family members.[17] An excerpt from the article follows:

"You be the husband and let me be the doctor." How many times have I heard this refrain? My usual response, spoken out loud or muttered under my breath, is "Right, if you'd be the doctor, I could be the husband." Where does the idea come from of completely dissociating the role of family member from that of physician family member? What is so improper about a physician being involved in the care of a loved one? Is it the potential for a clouding of judgment? No argument there: judgment is clouded, perspectives lost. But the issue is not that simple. What about the family doctor who is the only physician or one of a small number of doctors in a small town? What about emergency situations? Is the information provided by a physician family member necessarily wrong, distorted, suspect? Should it not be considered on its own merits?

How do responsible medical staff deal with the involved physician family member? Do they seek information? Do they invite him or her to be present at rounds? Do they allow or encourage the physician family member to see the patient's chart? Do they report investigations and lab results in general terms or provide the specific numerical results, or do they exclude the physician family member from the loop? What is the difference between giving feedback to a nonmedical family member in terms that he or she can understand and providing more technical feedback to a family member with a medical background? Isn't it just a question of providing information at the correct level for the specific recipient?

During the more than six months in three hospitals, I found Bonnie's care less than optimal on many occasions. The medical and nursing staff varied in their response to these discoveries. At times they were grateful for my intervention and responded with corrective measures. On other occasions some were angry and suggested that I was over involved and meddlesome. What I found most fascinating was that the staff who could deal with me were the best at their jobs, not only at the technical and diagnostic level but at the human level as well.

My experience only seems particularly strange because I am a doctor. What about family members who are not physicians? Are their ideas less valid? Are they less entitled to contest a dysfunctional system? I don't know if, as a physician, I had more or less difficulty in obtaining optimal care for my wife than a lay person might have had. Probably both. Considering my experiences, it is disturbing to consider how a non-physician family member could have dealt with the situation.

The irony is that anyone who has worked in an institution knows that mistakes are inevitable. People and machines are fallible, and in the end we need all the help we can get. Family members, physicians or not, need to be integrated into the care of a loved one. Their ideas must not be trivialized, their concerns demeaned. They, along with the professional staff, will have the best interests of the patient in mind.

Professionals need to work with the situation as it is. Information, from whatever source, needs to be weighed, taken seriously and put into context. Why should medical professionals check their training and experience at the door when a close family member gets sick?

Bonnie's book and my article opened an extensive discussion within medical circles. Bonnie and I were invited to present our story at several medical conferences, and many professionals, physicians, nurses, social workers and others wrote to me personally to present their own related role conflicts. The story triggered almost one hundred responses. It seemed that the struggle to work through the role as caregiver and professional hit a nerve. The stories came from physician children caring for parents, spouses caring for spouses, parents for children. Some were hilarious, but each story revealed a struggle.

In some stories it was clear that physicians had an inflated view of their skills, such that they insisted that they care for their own family members when others could easily have taken over the case. These physicians seemed to fail to appreciate the dire consequences for them and their family if they had taken on care for a spouse, child or parent and the outcome was poor or even resulted in death. Their arrogance is exactly why there are rules that require we do not care for our loved ones.

But in urgent situations where the physician is the only game in town, the rules can be a bit more flexible. My own engagement with my wife's care, and later my father's care, reflects a messy zone where the spouse or child is engaged with other caregivers who may or may not have the best skills or interests of the family member in mind. How you negotiate that minefield is an area for discussion. How to advocate for your family member when you are not a physician is a confusing zone. No one knows the family member better than you do. Your ideas need to be heard and weighed in the balance. Providers who understand this will probably provide the best care for the family members.

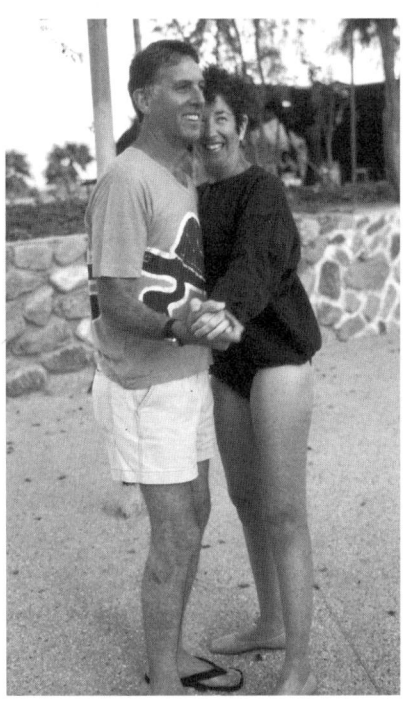

The cover photo from Bonnie's book *Slow Dance: A Story of Stroke, Love and Disability*. Although Bonnie could not stand on her own, when I held her we could slow dance. Bonnie's right brain gave her cues for weight shifts.

You may be wondering why I do not express more about how I was feeling during the many weeks of crisis when Bonnie was at death's door. I guess I wonder too. The answer is that I was in serious denial. The only way I could deal with the mess we were in was to become a fixer. I was always fixing stuff, offering work-arounds or alternative solutions, and collaborating with the nurses to improve care. I was in a state of constant vigilance, looking for omissions or mistakes in her care and stepping in whenever I thought something was going wrong. And as it happens, things did go wrong frequently, and under the supervision of the designated physicians and nurses, I even shared some of the care.

During Bonnie's care, I learned more about the role of alternative therapies in treatment, as I had not been exposed to such therapies in medical school. My first experience of working at the interface between Western and other types of treatments occurred in Chiapas, with the *curandero* healing ceremonies. One amazing example during Bonnie's long recovery occurred when our acupuncturist friend Bernard Côté wanted to do moxibustion to complement acupuncture. This involves heating a designated area with a cigar-shaped lighted tube filled with a smoking herbal substance, after which the area may be further treated with acupuncture. I had to temporarily surreptitiously disconnect the smoke detector in Bonnie's hospital room to allow this to happen. Bernard's treatment would cause Bonnie's drooping eyelids to go up like a window shade.

Subject to a variety of conventional and non-conventional rehabilitation modalities, Bonnie continued to improve, allowing her to have a productive life, despite her challenges. For the first time I appreciated the role of so-called soft therapies in patient management and began to send patients to selected acupuncturists for many diseases unsuccessfully

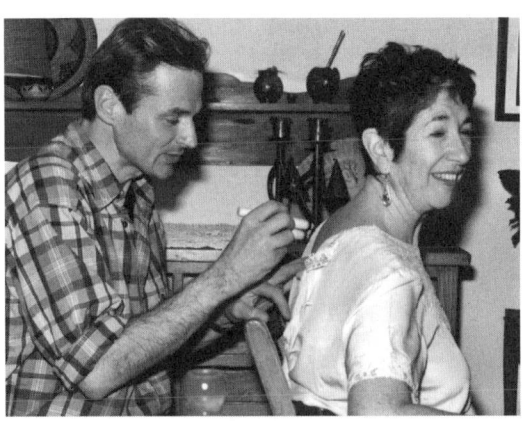

Our friend Bernard Côté, an acupuncturist, who helped Bonnie in many ways.

treated by Western methods, resulting in excellent outcomes. I became one of the few physicians in Canada to work regularly with acupuncturists, massage therapists and midwives. I always felt that we could use all the help we could get. In Montreal, we later established a pain clinic at the hospital where patients had the benefit of many medical and non-medical disciplines, all working together.

Several weeks after Bonnie's dramatic and life-saving surgery in London, she was deemed stable enough to return to Montreal for further treatment, and so off she went on the Quebec transport jet at no cost to us. Take note, Americans. We did have to pay for television rental.

One day, I was sitting in my office, taking a break from the neurological intensive care unit at the Jewish General Hospital, where Bonnie had returned for ongoing care. Suddenly, I heard a banging from the outer office. There

I saw a young rabbi affixing a mezuzah to the doorframe of my office. A mezuzah is a case that contains a small scroll inscribed with prayers central to Judaism, and it is a powerful symbol. Bonnie's situation was well known in the Jewish community. The rabbi was one of my patients, and he explained that he was concerned for Bonnie's health and wanted to provide all he could for her recovery. I thanked him for his concern. The mezuzah remained permanently—and who knows...?

One evening, as usual, I was sitting at the nursing station next to the neurological ICU. I was too preoccupied to see my own patients. I could not concentrate on their problems. Bonnie was no longer on a respirator, but she still had a tracheotomy in place. She was only able to be fed intravenously, and she was fed thicker, higher-protein fluids by a tube leading through her nose into her stomach. Suddenly, I heard Bonnie choking and ran into her room to see one of my patients, the religious father whose wife's birth I had assisted with over the touching issue. He was feeding her matzo, the dry crumbly unleavened bread Jews eat during Passover. She was choking and aspirating (down the wrong tube) into her airway and spewing matzo particles out of her tracheotomy tube. The nurse was momentarily out of the room. I quickly sucked out the crumbs and, enraged, chased the offender down the hall and out of the hospital.

The next day, my patient called to apologize. We had a strong relationship, and he apologetically explained that he had been trying to help. He had been feeding her a very special matzo, one that had been blessed the previous Passover by the chief North American Orthodox rabbi from Brooklyn, whom some of his followers believed was holy. I was not in a forgiving mood, though I eventually accepted his apology and we resumed a normal doctor-patient relationship, in which we were able to manage together some complex medical issues.

37. COMING HOME

BONNIE'S SERIES OF STROKES OCCURRED just as Seth, nineteen, was about to start at the University of Toronto. Well before her landmark surgery, a powerful moment happened after her second stroke, when Bonnie was in the ICU at the Jewish General Hospital, paralyzed in her arms and legs and unable to speak. Bonnie seemed agitated as I explained to her the confusion about Seth's imminent departure to begin his studies. Seth was conflicted about leaving Montreal, as he felt like he was abandoning Bonnie. I could tell that Bonnie wanted to communicate something. At first, I thought that, through a series of blinks, she was trying to indicate that she did not want him to leave. In extreme frustration, she managed to communicate that she actually wanted him to leave for Toronto, as she did not want to impede his education.

So Seth reluctantly left, but he began a regular pattern of taking the train from Toronto to Montreal every week. I would pick him up at the train station every Friday evening and return him to the station every Sunday night. There is no question that this pattern, though very helpful to Bonnie and the family in Montreal, interfered with Seth's ability to establish normal social relationships among his peers in Toronto. He later told us that he shared his mother's situation with very few of his classmates and new acquaintances.

Our daughter, Naomi, seventeen, was going through the usual adolescent struggles, particularly with me. Overnight, she left all that behind and became close to me, sharing the responsibility of visiting Bonnie and helping in many ways. Unfortunately, because of what I viewed as adolescent irresponsibility, I had not allowed Naomi to get her driver's licence when she turned sixteen. Now this decision came back to bite me. I really needed her to drive. A surgeon friend, Dr. Richard Margolese, asked me what many others were asking: "Is there anything I can do?" I replied: "Teach Naomi to drive." Within weeks, Naomi was driving.

Many people became close to Naomi and me during the worst time of Bonnie's illness. They offered what they could: taking care of our dog, making meals and providing many large and small acts of support. But a few could not handle such a severe illness and pulled away, never to be seen again. Some people that we hardly knew became close friends. One friend and practice colleague, Perle Feldman, memorably left a package at our door with a note: *When life is shitty, it might as well be shitty with chocolate chip cookies.* Some of Bonnie's friends engaged in healing ceremonies on Mount Royal.

Naomi was so deeply affected by Bonnie's strokes and complex recovery that she could not concentrate on her studies at Montreal's Collège Jean-de-Brébeuf. She stopped going to classes, dropped out for a year and spent her time helping me care for Bonnie. Despite trips every weekend from Toronto to Montreal to see Bonnie and help me, Seth thrived academically at the University of Toronto.

Misha, despite her need to focus on her studies in California, managed to come to Montreal several times when Bonnie was in the ICU. Having her with us was important for all of us. Her contributions included participating in healing rituals on Mount Royal with Bonnie's friends. Misha returned to her studies, went on to have much academic success, received her PhD in anthropology and became an academic anthropologist.

While Bonnie was hospitalized, I was too distracted to see patients or attend to my administrative duties as head of both the Herzl Family Practice Centre and the Department of Family Medicine at the Jewish General Hospital. I attended a few births, as it was enjoyable and therapeutic, but my colleagues took over the rest of my practice and the leadership of the centre. Cheryl Levitt became the acting director, a role that she filled extremely well. Later, she replaced me as head of the hospital department and the Herzl teaching centre when I left for British Columbia. Ultimately, she became the academic head of the McMaster University Department of Family Medicine. When we first met, she'd been a country GP on Salt Spring Island, one of the Gulf Islands near Vancouver Island. Michael Dworkind, an early resident and now staff, had recommended that I meet her. We three shared anti-war and environmentalist politics. Cheryl was a wonderful find as a practitioner and friend.

When I finally returned to practice, my nursing staff, Karen Tafler and Barbara North—who had always had expanded roles as nurse practitioners—were practising even more independently. For months, my patients seemed more concerned about me than themselves. They were extremely solicitous, presenting only their most serious problems. Karen and Barbara handled the patients with chronic conditions, routine well-child care and many new problems as well, knocking on my door to discuss only the most complex problems. This pattern had begun well before Bonnie's strokes, only intensifying after. Before the strokes, this pattern allowed me to have a full practice, even though as director I was officially practising only two half days per week. We had it organized so that, even when I was not scheduled to see patients, as my office was immediately adjacent to the offices of the nurses, they did not hesitate to knock on my door at any time to discuss concerns.

This pattern of working with the nurses had an interesting side effect. As the nurses were handling so many of the relatively straightforward practice issues, my own practice included only the most complex patients, the ones who took a great deal of time. I used to yearn for a simple ear infection or a routine case of adult-onset diabetes or hypertension, but I really had nothing to complain about.

As I returned to practice, patients often asked me how Bonnie's stroke affected me personally or psychologically. Did her illness make me a different person, perhaps a better person? I guess it did. I believe I became more attentive to the problems of others, and perhaps I was more sensitive and caring. Who knows? Though I like to believe I was this way before.

Bonnie's recovery was slow during the long rehabilitation phase. Eventually, she got to come home for weekends, with Naomi and me caring for her in familiar surroundings. It was an uplifting time. Bonnie worked at home with her film colleagues, editing the film *Mile Zero*, which she had shot just before her strokes. It was a film about Seth and three friends who founded an organization called SAGE, Students Against Global Extermination, to educate and mobilize high school students to prevent nuclear war.

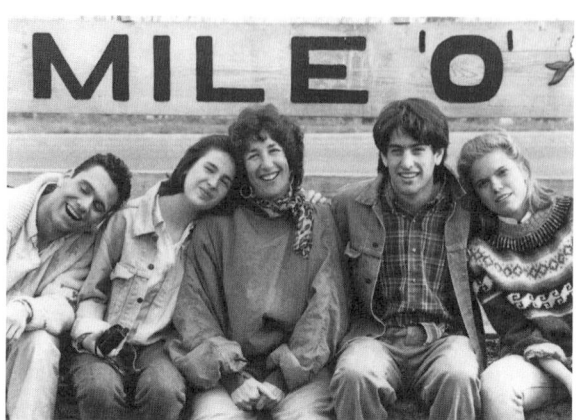

For a year, the SAGE kids crossed the country, from Newfoundland to Victoria, talking to one in twenty Canadian high school students. Bonnie caught up with them from time to time, documenting their experience. Part of Bonnie's rehabilitation was editing the film from home. But when Bonnie returned to the rehabilitation

Bonnie and the Students Against Global Extermination (SAGE) kids: (left to right) Max Faille, Desirée McGraw, Bonnie, Seth and Alison Carpenter during the filming of Bonnie's film *Mile Zero*, just before her stroke.

institute on Monday morning, tired from her editing, she was scolded by the occupational therapist for being too tired to make potholders. Get serious. Her weekend work *was* occupational therapy. Her occupation was filmmaking.

Did Bonnie's illness and long recovery affect our personal relationship, our marriage? Yes, it made us closer than ever. During the filming of *Shameless: The Art of Disability*, I was asked on camera why I had not left. In the face of profound illness, most men leave their wives. I at first joked, "Poverty of imagination," but after I got through laughing at my own joke, I said that Bonnie never changed. Sick as she was, Bonnie continued to be a positive part of the family. She continued to care for, and about, me and our children—even when she was paralyzed and confined to bed. Bonnie's positive outlook in the face of her illness and the many adaptations needed for her to continue to live a productive life was key. Her personality shone through, even during the period when she was the sickest and most disabled. To be honest, I imagine that if Bonnie had been a different sort of person, one with a negative personality, perhaps I would have left.

38. BACK PAIN

SEVERAL YEARS BEFORE BONNIE'S DRAMATIC illness, in the early 1980s, I injured my back, rupturing two discs, while playing squash. A chronic condition began that haunts me to the present. The discs were treated first with two levels of chymopapain, an agent long since discredited as an approach to disc rupture. In the end, I required complex and repeated back surgery, largely because of the use of this unfortunate agent.

Following the surgery, I had many months of severe back pain, eventually diagnosed as originating in destabilized facet joints. In desperation, I travelled to Cincinnati, where a special clinic provided what was then new, radiofrequency coagulation of the nerve endings of the facet joints from high in the lumbar region down to the sacrum, a procedure unavailable in Canada at the time. As in Bonnie's case, the cost was completely covered by Canadian Medicare.

The facet pain disappeared. But a new grinding pain was uncovered. Eventually, MRI studies showed that the end plates of the fifth lumbar and sacral vertebrae had eroded. It looked like the area had been eaten away, resembling Swiss cheese. The reason for this is unknown, but it was hypothesized that after the chymopapain got through "eating" away the offending discs, it continued on to eat the vertebral bodies. To escape from this pain, I was placed in a removable body cast from the thorax to low on my hips. In that state, for six months, I continued to practise and, within limits, even attend births.

In the end, finding a way to get out of the body cast was a major issue, finally aided by acupuncture delivered by our friend Bernard. Once I had escaped the cast, by word of mouth I collected a number of chronic back pain patients in my practice.

One memorable referral came via Bonnie, for an editor at the NFB. I made a house call to her Montreal East End apartment. Always looking for teaching opportunities, I brought along a young medical student, Vincent Lacroix, who was one of my advisees. The scene was stunning. The patient was on the first floor, where she had been for almost a year. Her husband and child lived on the floor above, the two floors connected by a spiral staircase. The patient had been suffering from severe back pain ever since the birth of her child, now a little more than a year old.

Mothering the child was impossible. The patient had a level of stiffness that was unique in its severity. She was in constant pain, immobile, depressed, suicidal and certain that she would never recover. The medical student became fully engaged with the family. In fact, he became a kind of godfather to the child.

We employed home physical therapy, massage, acupuncture and psychotherapy. As well, I used antidepressants and pain-relieving drugs. Who cares which treatment worked best? It was an emergency that required pulling out all the stops. Within a few weeks, there was major improvement, and within six months, the patient was mothering her child and back at work. The medical student went on to become a family practice resident and ultimately head of sports medicine at McGill.

Without telling me what she was going to do, the patient wound up on a popular CBC Radio talk show, where she told her story in four-part harmony, naming me and the medical student as her "saviours." The floodgates opened at the Herzl Family Practice Centre. A huge number of patients were calling, asking for appointments with me. Of course, all had severe back pain that interfered with their lives and employment. I could not handle the volume and had to develop a strategy. I instructed my secretary to say that my practice was full, *but* if the patients were willing to be seen by a first-year family practice resident (emphasize first-year), I would work with the resident in the provision of care. This screening manoeuvre reduced the number of patients to about twenty, all extremely pain-ridden and desperate.

I met with the residents and reassured them that each would receive only one such patient. I instructed them to begin each encounter with the following:

1. "I don't know how you have managed to deal with such severe pain for so long."
2. "I am sure that you have been told that it's all in your head. But it's in your back!"

After this opening, almost all the patients cried. At last, someone was listening. By this time, much of the pain was at least partially in their heads, in the sense that chronic pain always has a major psychological component. Nevertheless, the patients did not want to hear about their psychological state. Most patients come to a family doctor because they have conceptualized their pain as somatic, or physical, rather than psychological. It's the nature of our role.

After starting with those two opening statements, the residents could hardly believe their success with the patients. For all, we used multiple modalities, all at the same time. To everyone's surprise, almost all twenty patients improved in a major way, sixteen of the twenty returned to work and all but one made major improvements in their quality of life. Two patients were very special cases, which I took on myself.

Case 1: Mr. D. was a merchant seaman who was crushed against the side of the lifeboat and the hull of the ship in a Halifax lifeboat drill. He had been attempting for years to receive compensation from the company. He had been labelled a malingerer and even spent some time at the Allan Memorial psychiatric hospital in Montreal. I focused only on his somatic complaints. Central to my treatments were injections of the painful areas in his lower back.

At first, I used local anaesthetic agents with good success. Later, I used saline solutions, and then distilled water. Whatever I did worked, such that his visits were reduced to every three months. Usually, he would arrive bent over in apparent severe pain. He would leave upright and smiling. It was clear that there was a major psychological component to his pain.

One day, I received a phone call from his lawyer, who told me that I would soon receive a subpoena to appear in court. Why? Because the lawyer would use me to show that it was not in the patient's head after all. It was in his back, illustrated by my success in using physical not psychological modalities.

I explained that I would not be a good witness for his case, as to a large extent it was indeed in his head, but as the patient conceptualized his pain as physical, I treated the physical. The lawyer did not further engage me.

A few weeks before Bonnie and I were to leave Montreal for a new life in Vancouver, I was shopping in a nearby supermarket, where I clearly recognized my merchant seaman patient. He was smiling and chatting with people. His gait was fluid. He was upright and apparently healthy and pain free. I followed him surreptitiously as he did his shopping. No question, it was my patient. Should I confront him now or on his next visit? Do nothing? A week or so later, my patient appeared in the office in his usual pained and bent-over state. I decided that I had to say something.

"I can't help noting that I saw you in a supermarket and I was struck by how normal you looked. How is it that you looked so good then and you look so bad now?"

Smiling, he said, "Dr. Klein, I don't come to see you when I am feeling well."

Case 2: Ms. M. was a patient who presented with an unusual bent-over and twisted posture.

I asked, "Tell me, why are you walking like that?" to which she responded, "Like what?"

This is what Freud called *La belle indifférence*. It was classic for a conversion reaction, patients who convert their psychological symptoms into physical, often very bizarre, symptoms. A family practitioner can go their entire practice life and never see a conversion reaction; it is even very rare in psychiatric practice.

The patient was the sister of two of my patients and the daughter of an elderly man also in the practice. As this was such a complex psychiatric problem, I consulted Dr. Laurence Kirmayer, a friend and psychiatrist who was also an anthropologist and expert in transcultural psychiatry. We developed a program to delve deeply into the issues in the patient's life. We learned that she had suffered abuse at the hands of her father, my own patient!

Family practice could not be more complicated. Whole-family care can at times be both a blessing and a curse. Two of the three daughters had suffered the abuse, and the third was also my patient.

As we listened to her story, the abnormal posture seemed to unwind, and within several weeks she was standing erect, stating that a great weight had been lifted from her shoulders. Maintenance visits consolidated the gains, and she went back to work.

But what to do about the father? It turned out he had a serious cancer. Nevertheless, the daughters decided to confront their father and their mother, who they felt had failed to protect them from their abusing father. In a dramatic family conference, the daughters told their father what he had done to them and the profound effect his behaviour had on their lives. They were also able to express their confusion as to why their mother had not protected them. As their father slowly declined, he was able to acknowledge what he had done, and he deeply apologized for their pain and life disruption, leading to further improvement in the daughters' health. Just prior to his death, the daughters forgave him.

39. MAKING TROUBLE IN VANCOUVER

SEVERAL YEARS BEFORE I LEFT Montreal for a new position in Vancouver, I was invited to Vancouver to give a talk. I spoke about some of my research and how it can affect and lead to changes in practice. Later that day, there was a panel on birth. The panelists were a lawyer, an obstetrician, me and a woman (billed as "the consumer") who had experienced two births. She was the first to speak and told of her first birth, which she thought was horrible. She stated that her wishes and needs were ignored, and the birth was, in her opinion, unnecessarily traumatic. She described her second birth with a family practice colleague as wonderful. Her wishes were respected and she felt that her needs were discussed and acted upon.

At the end of her presentation, a very angry obstetrician in the audience attacked her as being interested only in herself and her experience. He stated that she did not care about the health of her newborn. He then said what she had done was tantamount to child abuse. The audience was shocked, hushed. I was due to talk next. I had prepared a detailed written contribution. Instead of giving my prepared talk I said, "Now you can see why women are having home births—anything to keep out of the clutches of a practitioner like this." I sat down. The audience went wild. Half supported me. The other half felt that I was rude and disrespectful. This event coloured the rest of the conference, with various proponents of different approaches to birth arguing among themselves and with me.

Two days later, my host drove me to the airport for my return to Montreal, still talking about the event. We were in the coffee shop when I noticed Margaret Atwood sitting at another table. I pointed her out to my host, who became excited and asked if I knew her. I explained that I had met her when Bonnie was making *Not a Love Story*. I said that she probably wouldn't remember me, and she looked tired and engaged with something. Under continued pressure, I finally agreed to say hello. She was friendly and invited us to sit with her. She immediately began, in her role as a curious reporter/novelist, to ask what I was doing in Vancouver. I told her that I had given a talk. She wanted to know more, so I told her the story about the panel. After a pause, she said: "I think you've got it wrong. It is you doctors who are the consumers. It is we women who are the providers."

I later learned that she was on a book tour for *The Handmaid's Tale*. When I later read the novel, I understood her interest in my story. The book describes a dystopia in which women are merely vessels for producing babies for the state. They have no rights and their children are taken away to be given to "more worthy" childless recipients. I think of Atwood's words when I see or hear of a birth that is fully "managed," when the woman is ignored and her contributions are dismissed. I hope that Atwood's look into the future does not happen. There has been some progress, but that type of experience, sadly, is not rare. Since the 2016 Trump election, *The Handmaid's Tale* has been reissued in hardcover and made into a TV series, its story more chilling and more prescient than ever.

40. LEAVING MONTREAL

Although Bonnie made a stunning recovery, she could not deal with Montreal winters. Operating a wheelchair or scooter in deep snow was impossible, and the snowplows obscured what curb cuts exist in that old city. Bonnie was indoors for up to six months every year. We had delayed moving to a warmer climate because I could not accept that Bonnie would never make a full recovery. I convinced myself that moving would be unnecessary. We loved Montreal, despite the endless linguistic wars and challenges for anglophones.

To delay making a decision about what to do to accommodate Bonnie's needs, I began a conversation with Richard Cruess, the same dean of medicine who bailed me out when I ran out of money for the episiotomy study. I explained that it looked like I would have to permanently leave Montreal and give up my academic and administration position and full tenure for Bonnie's well-being. We arrived at a compromise. For three to four months every year, during the worst of the winter, I would find work related to family practice in a warm climate.

As it happened, the McGill family medicine department had been asked to help Costa Rica establish its first family practice training program and they needed the first faculty. We were expected to teach the first trainees in

Spanish and then select some to be the first Costa Rican faculty. So Bonnie and I set off for Costa Rica, driving across Canada and the US on the way to Los Angeles, the point of departure. On the way, we stayed in Tucson with our old friends, the Ericksons.

All was well in Tucson, until I became seriously dizzy, so much so that it was even happening when I was lying down. It affected my balance too. I waited for it to resolve, assuming that it was a viral labyrinthitis, a temporary condition of the vestibular system. How could I drive to Los Angeles, especially when turning to the right triggered the dizziness? But I had to get there to begin the Costa Rican program. So I drove with my head either straight ahead or turning to the left while Bonnie surveyed everything on the right. It was as crazy as it sounds. We arrived in LA to stay at my brother's house. Then I called my classmate Peter Engel, who had helped me identify a surgeon for Bonnie.

On Peter's recommendation, I went to the dizziness clinic at UCLA. After a great number of neurological tests, the chief sat down with me and said, "Doctor Klein, you have had a stroke and you are not going to get better. And you cannot fly. You cannot go to Costa Rica."

Experts in denial, Bonnie and I flew to Costa Rica, with the dizziness continuing. I can't even remember why I did not accept the diagnosis. I just assumed that it would get better, whatever it was. So began a bizarre experience. As Bonnie drove her scooter, I would slowly walk alongside holding on to the left side of the backrest to prevent falling to the right. I taught in Spanish, carefully keeping my head forward. The condition slowly resolved over six weeks.

Clearly, I had not had a stroke. When I returned to California, I went again to the dizziness clinic, where the chief was not pleased to see me fully recovered; it seemed he would have preferred that his diagnosis was correct. I later learned that I have a temporary condition called benign paroxysmal positional vertigo, which still occurs infrequently.

Going to Costa Rica for two winters was perfect. We also went to Israel for two winters, with me as a visiting professor at Ben-Gurion University of the Negev. My role there was in faculty development. At the time, there were only fifty-eight Israeli academic family physicians and they needed instruction in their academic role. One of my activities was to bring the key Herzl/McGill family practice faculty to a development conference in Eilat, a lovely warm location on the Red Sea facing Syria, Egypt and Jordan and near the Sinai desert.

This led to a twinning of the departments of McGill Family Medicine and Ben-Gurion Family Medicine. We trained a faculty member from Ben-Gurion who later became the chair of family medicine at Ben-Gurion. In the process, I developed close personal relationships with a number of the first academic Israeli family doctors, many of whom served Arab and Bedouin villages and would be considered peaceniks.

It is worth remembering that the Herzl Family Practice Centre was named for Theodor Herzl, the founder of modern Zionism. These days there is serious conflict about the Israeli government's treatment of Palestinians. The Israeli occupation of the West Bank and the Gaza Strip and the relentless building of settlements on Palestinian land are making the creation of an independent Palestine almost impossible. Moreover, the incarceration of Palestinians in what amounts to a large jail in Gaza is hard to understand, given the history of anti-Semitism and the persecution of Jews during World War II.

When I left my role at Herzl in 1993 for our move to Vancouver, it was before the Second Intifada, or Palestinian uprising. Had I remained at the Jewish General Hospital, I would have been in continuous conflict with most of my colleagues, who justified Israeli government and military actions. Since the three Gaza wars, with the massive killing of Palestinian civilians, including many children, by the Israeli government and its military, I find myself deeply on the side of the Palestinians.

I struggled to run the family practice department from Costa Rica and Israel, with the evolving and unreliable internet in the early 1990s, but it eventually became impossible. So during a sabbatical in 1990–91, we began to look at alternatives on both sides of the border. Although job opportunities existed in warm parts of the US, it became increasingly clear that I could no longer accept the US model of care, which I had already experienced in Rochester—one system for the rich and upper middle class and another for the poor and sometimes employed. I was hooked on single-payer care, as we had in Canada, but nevertheless felt obligated to look in the warm parts of the US for potential jobs.

I considered the position of chair of family medicine at the University of California, Davis, which had a department with a good reputation. As part of my recruitment, but also a regular event, a drug company provided a sumptuous lunch. And I mean sumptuous: lobster, crab, exotic salads. I was expected to give a forty-five-minute talk on my episiotomy research.

Before my talk, the department arranged for a young drug representative to give her pitch about the latest—useless—non-steroidal anti-inflammatory drug. The audience uncritically allowed her to deliver absolute nonsense. Time went by. When she finished, I had twenty minutes left to give my talk. Turning to my audience, I explained that there was insufficient time for me to give the talk, which I declined to attempt. I expressed disappointment that an academic department would allow such a thing to happen. What kind of a model was this for the residents to see? What did that say about being an academic department? It was clear to me this was the wrong place for me. I withdrew from consideration for the position.

I was recruited to be head of family medicine at the University of Arizona in Tucson. After several days of meeting other department heads, it was clear that their notion of a department of family medicine was as a feeder for the specialists at the university. Not my idea of what I wanted to do with my life. After meeting many key department heads, I noticed that I had not been scheduled to meet the outgoing family medicine department chair. I pointed this out to the dean and asked him to set up a meeting. He reluctantly changed my schedule, and the outgoing chair picked me up for our dinner meeting—at his very own Italian restaurant. Without asking, he ordered for me. Our discussions quickly turned to the 1960s, when I had left the US for Canada. It was clear that he knew details about me that I had not provided. When I asked what he was doing during the 1960s and '70s, he responded, "I can't tell you. Classified. I will say that it was biological."

Then he told me, "Our family practice department has a contract with the US Navy. And if you get this job, our department will lose a multi-million, multi-year contract. You will never get clearance."

I was considering a job whose outgoing chair was doing biological warfare research! I learned that the ex-head had been kicked upstairs to an important position in the dean's office and would in a sense be my boss. Next morning, I met with the dean and withdrew my application. The dean was distraught, as he told me that he was about to offer me the job.

It was now clear to me that my professional future had to be in Canada, and there was only one city where the climate would suit Bonnie's needs, and the academic and practice setting would meet my needs. Carol Herbert, the head of the Department of Family Practice at the University of British Columbia, recruited me to head the family practice department at BC Children's and Women's Hospitals. The idea was for me to bring a non-academic department into the world of research. It was a marvellous opportunity, as Women's was both the tertiary maternity care centre for BC and the largest maternity care facility in Canada, with seven thousand births annually and, surprisingly, virtually almost no research. So Vancouver it was.

41. UNFINISHED BUSINESS

IT WAS TIME TO PREPARE for my departure from Montreal, where I had worked from 1975 to 1993. With the help of our nurse practitioners, I had conducted a full family practice, including all ages, and from about 1980 a large maternity practice. I wrote a letter to my patients, explaining that we were departing for a more forgiving climate because of Bonnie's needs. The patients all knew about Bonnie's illness and miraculous recovery. They were solicitous and at times embarrassed to be taking my time with "trivial" issues.

Because I explained that I really did not want to leave and expressed how much I would miss my patients and friends, it was very difficult for patients to be angry with me for leaving or say they felt abandoned, which is a common reaction among patients when their doctor leaves or retires.

As the departure date loomed, a series of almost incredible patient visits occurred. The common theme was patients taking the opportunity to finally conclude, manage or solve festering problems. For many patients, they were actually making a departure gift to me, a thank-you for the many times we had tried to solve problems together. Some problems that had seemed insoluble were now suddenly quickly resolved—as there was not much time left before my departure. Below is a sample of the many such patient encounters, some amusing, many tearful, some incredible—all powerful and indicative of patients' resilience and capacity for self-healing.

Case 1: Mrs. S. appeared in the doorway of the office a couple of weeks before my departure. She looked terrific. A woman in her seventies, she normally looked dishevelled and exhausted. Before I could say anything, before I could compliment her on how good she looked, she said, "I'm leaving that miserable SOB!"

I had been urging her to leave "that SOB" for many years. Her husband was a mean and abusive man who made Mrs. S.'s life miserable. The occasion of my departure provided Mrs. S. with the opportunity to finally take my advice. She made clear to me that this was her goodbye present. I was tearful and speechless.

Case 2: Within a couple of days, a similar event occurred. Mrs. A. stood in the doorway with her daughter and announced, "We are going to Florida. We have our tickets and are leaving tomorrow for a month's vacation."

Another present. Mr. A. had severe dementia and had not recognized her for many years. She was a devoted wife, and I had advised her to take time for herself and spend more time with her children and grandchildren. She assured me that this was the beginning of a new pattern. I told her how proud of her I was and how appreciative of the goodbye.

Case 3: I was at the meat counter in a local supermarket when a voice behind me said: "Dr. Klein, I am coming in for my six-week postpartum checkup."

"That's nice," I replied. "I look forward to it."

Mrs. B had been one of my most challenging patients. During each of her two pregnancies and before, pelvic examinations had been difficult for both of us, because of her extreme discomfort with the procedure, the only part of her examination that troubled her. During each of her two births, she had gone into a psychotic state, during which it had been impossible to communicate with her. It was her way of avoiding negative feelings that intruded on her consciousness. Early in our relationship, I expressed my view that women who responded to pelvic exams in this way (and of course had such a strong reaction during the births) had almost certainly been sexually abused. I asked her on several occasions if I was on to something. Yes, I was, she said, but she didn't want to talk about it. When I offered counselling with me or someone specializing in such experiences, she emphatically declined. I told her I was ready to discuss this further at any time.

The six-week postpartum checkup? It had actually been *a year and six weeks*. Mrs. B. appeared for her visit and internal exam and PAP test looking cheerful and relaxed. The internal exam went smoothly. What happened? "Dr. Klein, I took your advice and have been receiving counselling. Besides, you think you're getting away from me by moving to Vancouver? You forget. I work for the airlines and fly regularly to Vancouver. You're stuck with me." And so I was.

Case 4: I first met John when he was eight years old, having come into the practice with a diagnosis by a pediatrician of psychogenic abdominal pain, pain that is caused, increased or prolonged by mental, emotional or behavioural factors. It was soon clear to me that this unfortunate boy did not have psychogenic abdominal pain; he had Crohn's disease, a chronic remitting inflammatory condition of the small bowel of unknown cause.

John had a sardonic sense of humour even as an eight-year-old, and as he grew and developed it only intensified. John had all the complications and life-altering problems associated with the disease, the cause of which is still under debate.

As John aged, he had occasional bowel obstructions, some requiring abdominal surgery, as well as fistulas, rectal bleeding, et cetera. None of these complications were particular to John but just part of the disease. We had long and always amusing conversations about life and the unfairness of it all. John shared his troubles, loves and academic successes. He was admitted to McGill and graduated with honours, eventually deciding to be an accountant. I was gratified to meet his future wife, who became part of the practice, and I felt great pleasure at their marriage and pregnancy. I enjoyed being able to attend the birth of his son, such continuity always one of the high points of family practice.

John went to work for an accounting firm and soon had several exacerbations of his symptoms—and then some major complications. My problem was that I had several of the members of his firm in my practice. These patients had many psychosomatic and somatic illnesses that I could see were exacerbated by the work environment. It was the kind of workplace where the main partners were likely to be checking on their subordinates at 7 p.m.

to see if they were still working. The illnesses of the senior partners were not good for them, but they were disastrous for John.

I was in an awkward position because of confidentiality; nevertheless, I had to work on John's behalf. I was quite blunt with John. "You must get out of this workplace or you are going to die. Why don't you get a nice regular job with Revenue Canada? In any case, you must get out of this firm."

To my surprise, John followed my advice and got a nice nine-to-five job at Revenue Canada, probably reviewing my tax filing. His symptoms moderated. Instead of coming in for a final visit, he sent a letter:

> Dear Dr. Klein:
>
> So you are abandoning me. Not to worry. I know more about Crohn's disease than almost anyone on the planet—including you. I will manage my disease. I will teach Dr. Lorber [my replacement] all she needs to know about Crohn's.
>
> Get lost!
> John

It was typical of John, whose sardonic humour I had grown to appreciate. From time to time, I received a follow-up from Karen, my former nurse. John was doing as well as could be expected with Crohn's.

42. MY LAST
MONTREAL BIRTH

I HAD CARED FOR MRS. S. in her first pregnancy. During the birth, however, I was at a conference and covered by my able colleague Vania. Also in attendance was Mrs. S.'s not yet legalized midwife.

Mrs. S. had had an easy first birth in the hospital, resulting in many extremely positive memories. Now she was pregnant with her second; midwifery was still not regulated and she asked during a prenatal visit if she could have a home birth. She also asked what I thought about having her four-year-old daughter present at the birth. Her husband was adamant that home birth was out of the question: "Over my dead body." An unambiguous reaction.

I remember saying that at the age of four, attendance at a birth was not likely to be a request from the child, who would probably prefer to watch television. I inquired about what was motivating the request, and advised the parents that if they decided to have the child present, they needed to have another adult there to care for her, to determine if the experience was positive or negative and act as an interpreter for what was happening. Given the ease of the first birth and the questions being raised during the pregnancy, I decided to refer my patient to a not yet regulated midwife colleague for ongoing care, making myself available for shared care.

This went well until a few days before we relocated to Vancouver. We had moved into a temporary apartment downtown where late one evening I received a frantic phone call: "Come quick, the baby is coming!"

"Did you call the midwife?" I asked.

"Yes, she is here," the patient replied. "But please come quick. The baby is coming. My midwife is here, but she does not have her equipment with her."

"Did you call Urgences-santé [emergency services]?"

"Yes, but they are not here."

We lived only a few blocks from the patient's home. She lived in an unusual arrangement, with their shared architectural business on the first floor, living room on the second floor, kitchen on the third and the bedroom on the fourth. The home was one room wide with circular staircases connecting the floors.

It was snowing lightly. I quickly made my way to the home. I had no birth equipment, but I knew that Urgences-santé had emergency birth packs. I learned later that the midwife had not been expecting the birth and was not carrying her usual birth equipment in her car, including suction and oxygen. Hence, the need to call the paramedics. We needed their equipment rather than their help with the birth.

When I arrived, the baby was indeed coming. The head was crowning and the midwife was managing the birth. As I was washing my hands, the four-year-old was sitting on the end of the bed facing away from the birth, screaming "Be quiet, I am watching television!" In fact, she was watching *Beauty and the Beast*.

Just then, the paramedics arrived. The midwife borrowed the needed equipment, and together we sutured a small tear. We assured Urgences-santé that we had things under control, but they stayed until it was clear that all was well. They wanted to transport mother and baby to hospital, but we convinced them that it was foolish to transport a healthy mother and baby. We two would take responsibility. They left. In the meantime, the father was anything but elated.

"You did this on purpose," he accused his wife. "I did not agree to a home birth. I could be handing out cigars. Look at this mess."

The midwife and I were enjoying the scene to a certain extent, and we did our best to calm the situation. We obtained permission to call the grandparents, and one set quickly arrived, helped to settle the situation, looked after the four-year-old and started cooking. After a couple of hours, the situation in hand, I left. The midwife stayed.

During the next several years in my Vancouver office, I regularly received faxed pictures from a precocious girl as she grew up. When this young woman applied to McGill medical school, she asked me to write a letter of recommendation. As part of her application, she was required to write a story explaining why she wanted to be a doctor. She wrote of the story of her brother's birth, for which she claimed not to be present as she was out on the street with her father, flagging down a policeman. Moreover, she claimed that I got to her home too late and missed the birth. We had a fascinating conversation about perception. I later interviewed her, the mother, the father and the midwife about her brother's birth. All had somewhat different recollections of the event.

She got into McGill medical school and did well. Just prior to her acceptance, I had the pleasure of working with her on a research project about the attitudes of young people toward birth, a study that was published and remains a unique contribution to the birth literature.[18] She is now studying to be an internist-gastroenterologist.

43. BC WOMEN'S AND CHILDREN'S HOSPITALS

OUR ARRIVAL IN VANCOUVER WAS perfect. Wheelchair-accessible taxis were available everywhere, unlike in Montreal, where it was necessary to plan days in advance for a simple ride. From the airport to the city, no planning was needed. At last, Bonnie could be fully independent. Almost all buildings were accessible. Our reasons for moving were reinforced.

Professionally, however, Vancouver had a very different atmosphere from Montreal. Many members in my new Vancouver department thought of me as an intruder and "outside agitator." They had in mind a chief who was one of their own, someone local, who was interested mainly in financial and organizational issues, certainly not in research. The very idea of a chief of family practice interested in research and working with midwifery was insupportable for some. A small group of disgruntled members brought forward a motion to the hospital to have me impeached, citing that being head of a department of family practice and supporting midwifery were incompatible. The motion failed, but it became clear to me that I had a lot of work to do.

At the time of my arrival in Vancouver, BC Women's Hospital was not yet an entity. It was called Grace Hospital, and the Salvation Army ran it. The Salvation Army ran many small maternity hospitals across Canada. They were known for the excellence of their care, but it was difficult for them to run the only tertiary care maternity centre in BC. For the Salvation Army, another problem arose—the issue of abortion services.

Grace Hospital, Children's Hospital and Shaughnessy Hospital, a general hospital, were grouped together on the same site. The latter provided many services that supported the tertiary care mandate but also took Grace and the Salvation Army off the hook for abortion and other services that were uncomfortable for the religious order. But when Shaughnessy Hospital closed in 1993, just as I was arriving, it put Grace in some difficulty. How could a women's hospital not provide reproductive care services?

Within days of my arrival in Vancouver, a meeting was arranged between me and "the Major," the CEO of Grace. In full uniform, she said, "Dr. Klein, all I want to know is if you can support the mandate of the Salvation Army Grace Hospital." To which I replied: "I have spent almost twenty years as head of family practice at the Jewish General Hospital in Montreal. I think I can handle almost anything." That was the end of the interview.

It became increasingly clear, however, that although Grace ran a caring facility, the Salvation Army was not suited to run the tertiary care referral maternity centre for BC. Within a year of my arrival, the medical staff of Grace engaged in a full-scale revolt, demanding that the Salvation Army leave the hospital for it to become a real BC women's hospital. The Major and the Salvation Army departed, replaced by a secular administration.

Working in the largest maternity hospital in Canada afforded many opportunities. One of the early ones came when the administration asked me to support the evolving midwifery program. Midwifery was not yet legal in BC, but a group of midwives, educated mostly in other jurisdictions, were practising from the Women's Hospital base, without legal status. To support the midwives, I was delighted to put together a group of family doctors who would attend the midwifery prenatal clinic and be present on rotation for their births. It was good fun, but as the midwives were skilled, there was really not too much for us to do. I tried to stay out of their way, and to keep myself busy while attending births, I took many photographs and presented them to the couples.

On January 1, 1998, midwifery was fully integrated into the health care system in BC. Midwifery care was now fully covered in BC by the public purse. I've always been interested in transitions, so I placed myself on duty over the weekend when midwifery would transition into fully normal care, when one of our team would no longer have to be present for every birth. As the clock was approaching midnight, when midwifery would be legal, I was as usual in the room, taking pictures and trying to stay out of the way. It was 11:50 p.m. The baby was crowning. At 12:05 a.m. the baby was born. Turning to Camille Bush, the midwife in charge, I said, "Can I go home now?" "No, stay a while," she said. The baby needed a bit of care, which I did, but the midwives could have done it without me. They were trying to make me feel useful.

Before and after legalization, I was active on the Midwifery Implementation Committee of the provincial government, further inflaming some departmental members whose basic attitude was: "If the government is for it, it must be bad." My position has always been: "What do women need?" not "What do physicians need?" I never found promoting and defending family practice and supporting the development of both research in family practice and midwifery and woman-centred care to be incompatible.

Almost certainly because of my early life as an outsider, I have always identified with the underdog. Promoting family practice and full-service family practice maternity care, including delivery, fit nicely with a role that I relished. The struggle to promote family practice in its full potential for a society that needed it, when conventional forces were opposed, was a battle that I found invigorating. Being head of a department of family practice positioned me to take this on, and I was willing to accept the administrative part of the job to help make needed changes to maternity care.

I knew that regulated midwifery was needed, but I also realized that medical forces were bound to push against the movement. It had all begun back in Montreal, with the battle to integrate women's partners into birth. Putting myself in the centre of that revolution, first in Quebec and then in British Columbia, provided a focus for my need to improve maternity services for women and providers. As a departmental chair, I had the natural authority to address the naysayers. I used the actual data from my own Department of Family Practice, as well as conducting research that showed the safety of both family practice and midwifery, in and out of hospital. I doubt that I could have been as effective if I did not have the departmental platform from which to speak about what women and families needed for a movement promoting transformative birth.

As part of my Vancouver position, I also had a new role as head of outreach for the Children's Hospital. I tried to bring specialists to rural settings to save families long and expensive trips to Vancouver. When doing outreach to rural or regional settings, the specialists also ran educational sessions for the local practitioners. My most notable success was to bring cardiologists from out of the ivory tower to rural settings. The cardiologists loved it, as did the patients and the rural docs. As well, I established a First Nations advocate for Children's and Women's hospitals, a position that helped in a small way to ease the transition for a sick child or mother to a distant hospital from their rural or remote community. After a few successful years bringing specialists to local communities, the then CEO of Children's thought my ongoing outreach plan was too expensive, saying "Let them come to Children's." Since I was then unable to actually deliver an outreach program because the hospital resisted outreach, I quit that part of my job. There was still lots to do in my family practice role in both hospitals.

44. ANXIETY RULES

WHEN I TOOK OVER THE Department of Family Practice at Women's and Children's Hospitals in 1993, all of the 169 family physicians were attending births. When I left in 2003, fewer than half that number were attending births. Throughout BC, in the same period, the proportion of family physicians attending births dropped from 80 per cent to 30 per cent, while the actual number of family doctors attending births in BC dropped from 2,400 to about 800. And even this low number represented the highest proportion of family doctors attending births in Canada. In eastern Canada, the numbers have dropped much more precipitously—overall, only 11 per cent of family physicians attend births.

There are many reasons for family docs opting out of birth. They include the overproduction of obstetricians, the arrival of midwives (via a poorly thought-out provincial government financial package that made it appear, falsely, that the midwives were paid more than family doctors for similar activity) and regional health authorities closing small hospitals and putting in place regulations that are too unrealistic and restrictive to fit in with the many other things that regulating authorities expect family doctors to be competent in. As well, it is very difficult to integrate attending births and running an office.

As departmental head, at the same time that I was running programs to enhance family doctors' skills, I was faced with having to impose many restrictions on department members. The same thing was happening throughout the province. Many family doctors just gave up attending births, as they were told in many ways that delivering babies was a job best left to the experts— obstetricians. Moreover, it was common to diffuse the idea that even low-risk, healthy women could *frequently* get into trouble that could only be solved by obstetricians. Birth was increasingly seen as an opportunity for things to go wrong. Larry Reynolds, a family doctor in Winnipeg, was fond of describing the phenomenon by saying that increasingly women were seen as "unexploded bombs that needed to be defused."

It seemed that anxiety drove all decisions and actions, for both family physicians and obstetricians. Many of the new generation of mostly women obstetricians were increasingly planning never to experience vaginal birth themselves. You can imagine what they were counselling their patients. The problem is not that obstetricians are surgeons; they are, and we need good surgeons. The problem is that *normal birth has been turned over to surgeons*, when it ought to be in the hands of midwives and family physicians.[19]

In my role as head of the Women's Hospital Department of Family Practice, some physicians told me of their birth "war stories," frequently describing cases of shoulder dystocia, when the head is born, but the shoulders don't follow. Rapid resolution of this emergency requires the use of a series of specific manoeuvres. But other departmental physicians seemed never to have this problem. The answer to this discrepancy rested with the hospital maternity nurses, who told me that the physicians who often experienced shoulder dystocia actually caused the problem themselves because of their sense of urgency to deliver the baby before the baby underwent a normal rotation. Anxiety again! Working with some of these physicians resolved the problem. Others could not stop the behaviour, and most who could not control their anxiety gave up attending birth, which was probably a good thing.

Many problems in the department were resolved by confidentially giving the members their own rates of intervention—such as induction, Caesarean section, epidurals, episiotomy—so that they could compare their rates with their peers'. This comparison is best illustrated by the use of episiotomy rates, which were at about 45 per cent overall in 1995—some members had a rate of almost zero, whereas others had rates close to 100 per cent. After five years, the ones with the highest rates disappeared. Either they changed their behaviour or retired. In any case, the departmental rate fell to 12 per cent, and the severe trauma caused by overuse of episiotomy fell from 4.5 per cent to 1 per cent. Based on our own departmental data, we showed that members with the highest epidural rates also had the highest Caesarean section rates.[20] Thoughtful members began looking at their own rates and what to do about them. However, there were some holdouts who felt that their patients were more difficult or more neurotic or more demanding. There was no evidence that any of this was true.

At the same time that I was insisting that members study their own data and compare them to the departmental norms, I was also defending family doctors from attacks from specialists, who felt that those with low volume should retrain or stop maternity care. After careful study, we learned that the only difference between high and low volume family doctors was that the low-volume family doctors consulted with obstetricians more often and in so doing achieved the same outcomes as their high-volume colleagues. This research was published in the *Canadian Medical Association Journal*,[21] following which the Society of Obstetricians and Gynaecologists of Canada (SOGC) rescinded a policy statement that had urged low-volume physicians to retrain regularly, replacing it with an excellent position that careful *quality assurance* was actually what was needed. They urged that all providers be part of a program that would study outcomes regularly to assure the public that safety was being maintained. I had no difficulty supporting that position.

The reality is that family doctors have so many people looking over their shoulders in numerous settings, combined with obstetricians calling the shots, that their practice life is becoming overwhelming and for some unsustainable. At the same time, other social phenomena are conspiring to destabilize the maternity care system. The average age of obstetricians is fifty-eight. They are being replaced by mostly women obstetricians, who want a life outside work and often a reduced workload. If we don't rethink how we look after pregnant women, in the next ten years the maternity system will collapse. The good news is that in rural areas, obstetricians tend to be only consultants. They do not attend normal births because they are too busy with consultations from family doctors and midwives. This reality could force the development of a rational and sustainable model for the whole maternity system.

Fortunately, at the University of British Columbia there is a renaissance of family doctors attending births, with up to 50 per cent of graduating residents deciding to incorporate maternity care and birth into their future practice, and much higher rates among our residents planning a rural practice. Why at UBC and not elsewhere? It is because in all our training settings, we can show our trainees that this work can be done without destroying your life or your marriage, or stressing your kids. We have shown that hard call produces enough volume so that the family doctor on call can be busy attending their own patients and those of the group.

As we did with the birth team we developed in Montreal, we started meet-the-doctor nights at Women's on the Family Practice Maternity Service, where we consciously demonstrated our common philosophy as we took turns answering questions. These evening sessions every few months for a couple of hours allow the couples approaching the time of their birth to meet all the members of the birth team. Couples see that they are better off with someone they have maybe just met rather than their own doctor, who might be exhausted and distracted at the time of the birth. As one of the founders of the Family Practice Maternity Service at BC Women's, I took my turn covering all the members of the seven-doctor group. Family practice maternity services, organized to provide care for the patients of family docs who do not attend deliveries, were popping up all over BC and other parts of Canada.

Covering other family physicians' patients was almost as much fun as attending my own. One night when I was on duty, I entered the room of a patient and her partner, both women. The labouring woman's mother was also present. I introduced myself. "Oh, we remember you from meet-the-doctor night. Welcome to our birth." I indeed felt welcome. The labouring woman was directing her mother to take videos of the labour and birth, providing very specific instructions as to what to shoot and when.

After I had established a relationship, I gently reminded them that, as they knew, this was a teaching hospital. I explained that the medical student on duty, as with all the medical students at the time, had never been present at a normal birth. They had only been at complicated births, often with forceps or a Caesarean. Sadly, the students had never seen the kind of birth that I predicted these women were going to have. The new parents seemed open to having a medical student. "There is only one potential issue," I explained: "All the med students on duty today, as it turns out, are male." Short pause.

"Bring him on!" The student was more than six feet tall, with big hands. He did a lovely delivery, with my hands on his hands, while I whispered in his ear what to do. With the baby born and on the mother's chest, the student began to sob uncontrollably, finally saying what a beautiful experience it was. Even though he planned to be a neurosurgeon, he was especially appreciative of the experience, as he planned to be a father in the future and wanted to be part of such a birth.

He could not stop talking about the birth to his fellow medical students, several of whom demanded the opportunity to experience the same kind of birth. They did so with family doctors, a few midwives and the occasional obstetrician. Some of the students declared that they were more interested in attending normal births than a session in the urogynecology clinic, where most of the women had urinary incontinence and where students, and even future obstetricians, easily get the idea that birth is only an opportunity to develop pelvic floor problems. This distorted view of birth is a defect in training at all levels.

Obstetricians are taking the hard call, or group approach, as well, with some having a coverage group member who stays at the hospital, but there may not be the same common approach among their coverage groups. The first generation of midwives believed in complete continuity of care until death or divorce. The new generation of midwives were exposed to the shared hard call model early in their training, so they also tend to practise in groups. Burnout does nobody any good.

In BC, and more so in other jurisdictions, as the system collapses under inadequate numbers of birth providers, ministries of health and education must work together to plan what kind of system the province needs. How many obstetricians, and where ought they to practise? How many family doctors doing maternity care, and how many midwives? Where should they be educated, by whom and in what educational environment should the right practice messages be delivered? Then they will have the opportunity to design a rational system that serves women and families, while improving practice for the professionals as well.

45. ORGANIZATIONAL SHENANIGANS 101

ABOUT FIVE YEARS AFTER MY arrival in Vancouver, and after many organizational changes, yet another new president for Women's and Children's arrived from Montreal, still one of the most specialist-dominated cities in Canada. Shortly after her arrival, I was invited into her office.

"Dr. Klein, your department is too large [it was 169 members] and the budget to care for them is too large. This is *the* tertiary high-risk referral centre for the province. I don't understand the role of general practice," she said.

I explained that only about 15 per cent of the seven thousand births in the hospital every year were high risk; the rest represented average women from the community—just having a baby.

"I want you to cut the size of your department in half," she said. We were by far the largest department in the hospital.

Unable to resist, I replied: "You mean that if we had fewer family doctors on staff, women would have fewer babies?"

On top of that, she said: "I cannot understand why GPs should attend their child patients in our pediatric emergency room."

Flabbergasted and fearful that I was going to say something I would regret, I made some sort of excuse to leave the interview.

Shortly after, without preamble, our new CEO appeared at the Medical Advisory Committee, where every department head sits, and said: "I cannot understand why a tertiary care centre has a Department of Family Practice sitting on this committee."

After a stunned silence, the head of psychiatry, in a memorable moment, asked, "Are you crazy?" She did not last long. She went back to Montreal.

We had so many changes in leadership in a short time that I stopped orienting the next one, as it seemed that they would not be here long enough to make such activity useful. I called them "temp CEOs." They came in, changed the mission, shuffled organizational models, cut the budget, fired some staff and left with a good departure financial package, then moved on to denude the next organization.

These administrative and organizational issues are unavoidable. If I was going to be silly enough to continue to head up a department, I would just have to put up with it. For one's sanity, however, it is important to realize that all organizations behave this way. Organizations have no memory, or it is a rare one that does. Professionals working in large organizations have to know that continuous organizational change is the norm. Organizational loyalty is a myth. So when the new CEO enters the scene and tries to put their personal stamp on the organization, they will make many changes, most of which will not improve the situation, and many of which will make it worse. The stationery manufacturers benefit, as the latest logo or mission statement is part of rebranding the organization, but the staff will do well not to take it too seriously.

That said, it's clear that being a department head can be a stressful and often thankless role. At times, I considered removing myself from all that conflict, but I also thought seriously about how that would affect my ability to make change—so I hung in. The Rochester experience may have influenced me, as I discovered the downside of giving up control.

46. "TOO POSH TO PUSH"

As THE CARE OF WOMEN in childbirth has increasingly moved into the hands of obstetricians, the landscape has continued to change. Caesarean section is increasingly used as the solution to most problems, real or imagined, while the skill set to attend birth with forceps or approach vaginal breech births atrophies. Perhaps most alarmingly, birth has come to be feared, not just by the general public but by obstetricians and other birth attendants.

This trend is easy to understand. At the level of training, future obstetricians are little exposed to normal birth, but they spend a great deal of training on the pathological. Moreover, they spend no time with the evolving generation of regulated midwives. Family doctors are caught in the middle, having been taught by obstetricians that the field is better left to the experts and that attending birth is hard on office practice, not to mention the long hours, both day and night.

The rise of Caesarean section on demand became one of the foci for my ongoing research on birth attitudes of both the caregivers and women.[22] It was an interesting dance between maternal autonomy, including the right to elective Caesarean, and doing the right thing in practice. The two concepts collided, with one school feeling that modern women, with their increasingly complex lives, had the right to decide on their mode of birth, even if there were no obvious indications for a Caesarean for themselves or their fetus—and even if their choice was more dangerous for themselves or their fetus.

The move to more general acceptance of Caesarean section as just another way to have a baby is illustrated by the comment of an old obstetrician colleague: "You know, Michael, it hurts me to have to admit that your study really did show that episiotomy does not do what we thought it did. But you know what the real problem is? *It's vaginal childbirth itself!*" At the time, I actually missed the point. At first I thought that it was good news that he acknowledged our research showing that episiotomy should be limited. But it was not long before I realized that vaginal childbirth was coming under attack.

As more and more obstetricians were becoming comfortable with Caesarean section to resolve increasing numbers of the presumed abnormalities of childbirth, many policymakers and the public were asking what had changed to lead to an increase in Caesarean rates from 3 per cent to 5 per cent in the 1950s to around 30 per cent at the end of the twentieth century.

The surgical approach of obstetricians is not at all surprising—they are surgeons. But pro-Caesarean biases begin early. When I surveyed obstetrical residents about why they chose to train as specialists in OB/GYN, 82 per cent indicated that it was the surgery that motivated them. When asked what they liked least, they replied: "Being with women in labour." They saw that as somebody else's job. Women's health was not even on their radar. If obstetricians in their professional and personal lives are now governed by fear of childbirth, we as a society have to help them get over their fears, while at the same time addressing our own fears of childbirth.

North American obstetricians are even more inclined than UK or Scandinavian obstetricians to accept Caesarean section by choice, but whose choice? The issue is confounded by the growing trend to support women's autonomy, such that the two issues are at war with each other. Female and younger obstetricians are more inclined to emphasize autonomy but are more fearful of bladder and sexual dysfunction after their own birth—this, even though overall maternal and perinatal mortality, and short- and long-term maternal and neonatal outcomes, favour vaginal delivery, with credible research showing that by six months post-delivery by any mode of birth, there is little difference in sexual functioning.

One of the wonderful anomalies in this discussion on mode of birth was that almost all Scottish female consultant obstetricians were selecting vaginal birth for themselves. Moreover, those who had experienced vaginal childbirth would have nothing else. This view, compared to their London female colleagues doing the same job, is fascinating. Guess it is time to go to Scotland to find out why.

In Canada, the SOGC is clear that vaginal birth is the preferred and safest route in first and subsequent pregnancies for mother and fetus. Nevertheless, it may be difficult to resist a request for Caesarean even if it seems unreasonable, as agreeing to it respects the views of women and the increasing complexities of their lives.

Focusing on the obstetricians alone neglects the role of women in society, and the influences all around them. Normal childbirth has become jeopardized by inexorably rising interventions around the world. In many countries and settings, Caesarean surgery, labour induction and epidural analgesia continue to increase beyond all precedent, and without convincing evidence that these actions result in improved outcomes. Use of electronic fetal monitoring is endemic, despite evidence of its ineffectiveness and negative consequences for most women when used routinely. In fact, routine use of electronic fetal monitoring only increases the Caesarean section rate, without helping the fetus, unless the fetus is clearly in severe distress. Even then it is unreliable technology, as what we really want to know is what is going on in the fetal brain, but we measure the fetal heart rate. No wonder we get it wrong so often.

Despite increasing appreciation of the need for evidence to govern practice, episiotomies are still routine in many settings despite clear evidence of their danger when used indiscriminately. Many other medical procedures that have been disproven in studies—un-physiological positions for labour and birth, pubic shaving and enemas, routine intravenous lines, enforced fasting, overuse of drugs and early mother-infant separation—are still used regularly in some settings.

Unfortunately, our research has shown that family-centred maternity care can only have a limited effect if the system is designed to remove women from their own decision making. The midwifery contribution to improved outcomes, in my opinion, is to a great extent based on the midwives' ability to keep women out of hospital until women are in active labour. Doulas (birth coaches) can also keep women out of hospital until they are in well-established labour. Keeping women out of hospital to a large extent mitigates the anxiety of both staff and women that is so central to the medicalization of childbirth and the increasing rates of Caesarean section and other procedures. Our research has shown that various methods used by the hospitals to delay admission until labour is established have all failed to demonstrate reduction in procedures and Caesareans. Although they're important, these are small interventions compared to the large intervention of having a midwife or a doula. Our research has demonstrated that once women come to hospital early, before the onset of active labour, they seem doomed to care in a rigid institutional system where anxiety over potential problems undermines maternal confidence and leads to a self-fulfilling prophecy.

Why aren't more women complaining? Because we are a terrified, risk-averse society, and birth is no more immune to the societal trend to "Ask your doctor for…" something for your high cholesterol, arthritis, thinning hair, facial wrinkles or lousy sex life. Pop a pill and carry on being fat and out of shape, then die suddenly at age ninety in the middle of sex.

We demand perfection of society, the medical profession and ourselves. Meanwhile, women—more and more often pregnant for the first time at thirty-five to forty years of age, with a profession and infertility problems because of delayed childbearing—are asking for a pre-emptive Caesarean section despite no indications for themselves or their fetus. Unsupported, induced, monitored, epiduralized, vacuumed, forcepped and ultimately C-sectioned—and all within an environment hostile to vaginal birth.

Recent studies have contributed to this dystopic birth environment: the post-term induction study and studies of vaginal birth versus Caesarean section for breech babies are good examples of research that changed practice so that important professional skill sets were lost, while mindless inductions clutter up the birth suites to the detriment of women in spontaneous labour. These destructive changes happened because we let them happen.

Society's fear of birth in the early 1920s, during Dr. DeLee's time, was based on the actual experience of negative outcomes. Fear was logical, as both mothers and babies were indeed dying. Thus, at the time, it seemed reasonable to cede control to surgeons, who routinely employed episiotomy and outlet forceps. Later, when safer Caesarean sections became available, they began to use the procedure more regularly to solve the very real problems of childbirth at the time.

As a society, we want to believe that all problems can be predicted and prevented. When perfection fails to happen, patients and their families take it out primarily on obstetricians, legally mostly, but in many other ways too. A famous obstetrician summed it up: "When you want to play God, don't be surprised if you are blamed for natural disasters." Women and their partners go along with this stuff because they are afraid, and many believe, falsely, that the "perfect" child will be born by elective Caesarean section. Women also often lack knowledge of the options available to them. The most risk averse of them select obstetricians for normal pregnancy and birth. The least risk averse select midwives for home birth and those in between want a midwife and an epidural. These select hospital birth with a midwife or a like-minded family doctor. And those who are confused or uninformed, or have no choice—or love their family doctor—choose a family doctor. In the end, everyone is happy in their niche-market world.

47. ATTITUDES TRUMP EVIDENCE

BEFORE EPIDURALS WERE READILY AVAILABLE, skilled maternity nurses employed a wide range of techniques to help women with the pain of labour, while managing their charting and the equipment, including IVs and the newly available electronic fetal monitors. With the advent of routine epidural analgesia, things began to dramatically change. More and more women were demanding epidurals, and across North America, dedicated epidural services were developing, especially in high-volume birth settings. In many such settings, anaesthesiologists were on salary to provide twenty-four-hour service.

As routine epidurals became available, the skill set of the maternity nurses changed. Experienced labour nurses retired, and their younger counterparts were more engaged with managing the equipment that was then required for safety reasons when epidurals were in use, distracting nurses from their traditional role of hands-on support for the labouring woman. In one key study, it was shown that only 15 per cent of a maternity nurse's time was spent "hands on" with the women under their care. The rest was spent on the equipment, charting and the many demands placed on nurses by the institutions for which they worked. Many nurses appreciated the tension between what they knew they should be doing and what they had to do for the job, and they were not happy about it.

When doulas appeared in the 1990s, they began to take on some of the intimate caring that had previously been the role of the maternity nurses. Some nurses were at first resentful of the doulas, but with time, nurses came to appreciate the complementary nature of the nurse-doula role. An important study showed that maternity nurses could not function as doulas, even when trained to do so. This was because the nurses, no matter how motivated to provide the intimate maternal care needed, had primary responsibility to the hospital, whereas doulas had primary allegiance to the woman.

Meanwhile, across the world, epidural research was developing, run mainly by anaesthesiologists, who investigated the role of epidurals in Caesareans and other procedures. The typical RCT compared epidurals against narcotics. There have been no studies that compare epidurals against physiological techniques, or physician births versus midwife births. Nevertheless, the "scientific" community managed to convince themselves, most of the medical community and many women that *routine* epidurals did not have negative consequences.

Of course epidurals have many positive attributes, especially when used *selectively* to problem solve, but many of us could see the negative effects when they were used routinely, without thought for consequences. This was vigorously denied by the anaesthesia community, which over time had developed a deep attachment to the procedure, especially as dedicated anaesthesia services had developed specifically around the provision of epidural analgesia for labouring women. Anaesthesiologists, using the new scientific approach to birth, learned how to design the studies that would give them the answers they sought.

Some of us knew that other methodologies beyond the RCT would have to be used to understand the full effect of epidurals on the birth environment. My first epidural study compared births as managed by high-volume versus low-volume epidural users in my own department at BC Women's. It demonstrated that the high epidural users had much higher Caesarean section rates than the low epidural users. Moreover, the high users had more newborn complications as well.[23] Next we compared epidural use at BC Women's with a nearby community hospital. When we controlled for all the relevant variables, it was clear that epidurals increased the Caesarean section rate threefold.[24] Then I looked more deeply at the evidence that indicated epidurals had no effect on various procedure rates. To do this, I separated the studies that used epidurals after labour was well established (when epidurals should ideally be used) from those that employed epidurals early in labour. When I eliminated the studies that appropriately used epidurals late in the birth process, I was able to demonstrate that early epidurals more than doubled Caesarean section rates.[25]

The anaesthesia community greeted these studies with outright derision. Only their own RCTs mattered. In fact, what mattered was how the epidural was used and under what conditions. The problem with almost all the studies that claim epidurals had no effect is that they took place in tightly controlled settings that did not approximate clinical reality. Moreover, epidural use cannot be separated from the whole range of interventions that characterize birth today. There is only one study that has shown that in a low Caesarean environment, epidural analgesia done early in labour will not increase the Caesarean section rate. This is because in that study environment, nurses and staff were using a variety of methods to help women with their labour pain. Epidurals were only one of the tools that they used. In such an environment, the staff do not use epidurals routinely as the solution to most problems. When birth attendants use epidurals selectively, the epidural either does not have the usual negative effect, or even has a positive effect (with no increase in Caesareans, or, rarely, a decrease). Many conventional practitioners and the anaesthesia community either don't know about or dismiss this information.

What is needed is right-brained thinking, or seeing the whole picture, for any procedure, both for the first time it is used and the implications for its potential repeated use. This is best exemplified by the way a Caesarean sets the scene for a cascade of negative outcomes for mother and baby in subsequent pregnancies, leading to placental attachment problems, infertility, ectopic pregnancy and stillbirth. The problem is that trying to avoid stillbirth, through frequent use of induction of labour in late pregnancy, paradoxically results in an excess of stillbirths in subsequent pregnancies.

Sadly, with the overuse of Caesarean sections and the current obesity epidemic with resultant diabetes, for the first time, the maternal mortality rate in BC, since 2014 through 2018, has risen rather than dropped, increasing from 3 per 100,000 to 5 per 100,000. In some jurisdictions of the US, maternal mortality in 2017 reached 18 per 100,000—some because of the overuse of Caesarean section. As of July 2017, President Trump and the Republican-dominated US House of Representatives and Senate are trying to remove health care from between 21 million and 32 million Americans. This strategy includes defunding Planned Parenthood and making drastic cuts to Medicaid, which funds almost half of all births in the US. They also plan to deny coverage for vaginal birth after Caesarean (VBAC) because it is a "pre-existing condition." These draconian cuts, designed to free up funds for a tax cut for the uber rich will result in a further dramatic increase in maternal mortality.

To understand the role of attitudes in maternity practice in a scientific manner, I launched a funded national study of attitudes and beliefs of the full spectrum of providers of maternity care: obstetricians, family physicians, midwives, obstetrical nurses, doulas and the women they serve.

In some respects, the results were no surprise. In other ways, they were illuminating. It was clear that most obstetricians were deeply attached to Caesarean section, 20 per cent failing to appreciate that it was not as safe for the mother or fetus than a planned vaginal birth. Many in the new generation also did not appreciate that epidural analgesia had transformed birth in Canada, sometimes for the better and sometimes not. The older obstetricians knew the negative effects of epidurals as well as the positive, as they had been in practice when epidurals transformed birth. The younger obstetricians could not see the change because they had grown up in an epidural environment.[26]

The younger obstetricians, 82 per cent of whom were women, were the most likely to employ epidurals, Caesarean section and some other procedures. They were also less likely to feel that the woman had a significant role in her own birth than their older, usually male colleagues. Many were planning never to experience vaginal birth, because of their fears of urinary incontinence and pelvic floor and sexual dysfunction. Importantly, it was not a *gender* issue, as the 18 per cent of male obstetricians in the study felt the same; it was a *training* issue.

Although obstetricians were generally supportive of midwives—less so doulas—they were deeply distrustful of home birth and other out-of-hospital birth settings. In many respects, these attitudes were not surprising, as they had been exposed in their training only to high-risk situations—never spending any time with midwives or training on the normal situations. Their only exposure to home birth occurred when a labouring woman was transferred to hospital with a problem. Most of the time, it was only for further pain management, but obstetricians-in-training focused on the rare negative outcomes, failing to appreciate the positive.

The idea that obstetricians supported midwives but distrusted home birth, almost half of what midwives did in practice, demonstrated how critically important it is to look for opportunities for obstetricians to work with midwives, particularly during training.

Our study highlighted that opportunity for collaboration between several birth-related disciplines certainly exists, as we found that 20 per cent of obstetricians had attitudes and beliefs that were similar to those of midwives. Our study also demonstrated that most obstetricians and some family physicians believed that the majority of women should be encouraged to receive routine epidural anaesthesia. Many failed to appreciate the connection between routine epidural analgesia use and an increase in forceps, Caesarean section and other interventions. Insufficient numbers of practitioners appreciated that even the first Caesarean can lead to known problems in placental attachment in subsequent pregnancies.

Although I focused earlier on the central role of obstetricians in the evolving birth crisis, my discipline has its own problems. We found that the new generation of family doctors who were delivering babies were progressive and appropriately positive in their attitudes toward childbirth, but those family physicians who were not delivering babies were, for the most part, still providing antenatal care. In fact, more than 50 per cent of the antenatal care in Canada is delivered by family physicians who did not attend the actual birth. Their attitudes toward birth were often negative or frankly wrong, and these attitudes began when they were in training.

What was disturbing was that family physicians who didn't attend births were in a position to expose their patients to their negative attitudes before transferring them, usually to an obstetrician, for the actual delivery.[27] Since so many family doctors practise only antenatal care and have problematic attitudes, we family doctors need to arrange courses to help those doctors acquire and maintain attitudes, knowledge and beliefs that are correct and supportive of normal vaginal childbirth, even if they themselves do not attend births. I am pleased to say that such courses are now beginning to be offered.

The good news from my perspective is that a significant number of obstetricians in our study would have preferred to work only as consultants to family physicians and midwives rather than practise first contact OB/GYN. These obstetricians are the natural allies of both midwives and family doctors and represent hope for a more rational future. Although the professionals have a great deal to account for, to blame them completely is unfair. Women and families are often willing participants in today's dystopic birth environment. It is unreasonable to expect health professionals, on their own, to change the attitudinal environment of birth.

Solutions to the accelerating birth crisis will require pressure from women, as was the case in the 1960s, '70s and early '80s, when hospitals were forced to open up births to partners, improve the physical setting (birth rooms and single-room maternity care) and reduce or eliminate harmful practices like routine shaving, enemas and episiotomy. This led to what we now call family-centred maternity care, which now includes early skin-to-skin contact between mother and newborn, universal rooming-in and the demise of central nurseries, on-demand breastfeeding and doulas to mother the mother. Dr. Marshall Klaus was responsible for many of these positive changes, changes that flowed directly from his research on bonding and attachment and the role of a supportive companion (doula). Today, for the needed change to happen, in what might be called a new birth revolution, women need to be educated about truly *evidence-based* maternity care.

We know from our national parallel study of women approaching their first birth that most, even late in pregnancy, are unclear about issues that are fundamental to the birth process.[28] Most do not take prenatal classes, and many get their information from the deeply flawed internet. Childbirth education should not teach compliance with a flawed system but rather be evidence-based and woman-centred, not institution-centred. Our study showed that, depending on the issue (Caesarean, episiotomy, induction), 30 per cent to 50 per cent of women, even late in pregnancy, are unsure of these critical issues and therefore unprepared to express their concerns and enter into a dialogue with their chosen provider. And if 20 per cent of obstetricians have misinformation about these same issues, we can see how problematic a discussion might be between an uninformed woman and a misinformed birth provider.

As the issues are so pervasive, I am afraid that minor alterations will not fix the system. The educational and delivery system for women requires a complete refit. I hope to be around to at least see the process begin.

48. RURAL MATERNITY CARE

INCREASINGLY, WOMEN AND THEIR FAMILIES have to travel sometimes hundreds of kilometres to access quality maternity care. This travel puts tremendous strain on expectant mothers, their families and their communities, particularly in rural and Indigenous communities, where the shortage of maternity care is experienced most acutely. We know that when women have to leave their communities to receive essential maternity care, they are under increased stress, and health risks and adverse outcomes increase for both mother and baby, even when excellent care is finally provided in distant locations, leading to increased costs to families and the provincial health care system.[29]

Over the past twenty years, especially in rural settings, regional health authorities have relentlessly closed small maternity units. They claim such units are either too small to be safe or not economically viable, or both. The actual data shows that such units, at least in western Canada, have been shown to be safe—surprisingly, even some without immediate Caesarean section capability. This is possible because the staff at such units easily transfer high-risk women to higher levels of care before or during labour, and because they transfer early, when problems are developing—and because medical and nursing staff are determined to keep their skills up to date. Also, hospitals that receive these needed transfers from another hospital or a home birth in progress are positive in their role.

Throughout my career I have worked with local, usually rural, communities to help keep their maternity services running. It was always a politically dangerous activity, as the regional health authorities were never happy with my intervention. It has been a struggle, as the trend is for local authorities to eliminate those services, merely to save money, even when they are functioning well and have excellent safety outcomes for mother and baby. We joke that the perfect Canadian hospital has no beds, no staff and no patients. The budget is balanced every time.

When I was evaluating maternity services in northern BC communities, I also found good examples of physicians committed to those communities in which they lived. The United Church of Canada was responsible for the medical care in several northern BC communities where all the doctors were on salary. A few other communities ran with what is called alternative payments, in which all staff including doctors are on salary. Long-term stability has been achieved because doctors and all staff have the time and the needed organization to focus on the needs of their community rather than worrying about their financial requirements. Team practice is the norm. The needs of patients and the community are addressed in a collaborative enterprise. The doctors, nurses, nurse practitioners, public health nurses and others meet regularly to develop policy, plan individual patient care and think of how they can address community health issues.

Some remote locations have so few births that maintaining an unsustainable service makes no sense. But we are in a time when loss of maternity services from well-functioning units serving their communities is actually dangerous for the women who have to travel long distances to receive service. And it costs them and their families substantial dollars to uproot themselves and pay for travel costs, lost wages for the partner and support services like babysitting.

Moreover, the data shows that when healthy, low-risk women have to travel long distances to give birth to an average-sized baby, the results are less good than if they stayed in their home community. There are many reasons for this, chief among them the loss of support during labour and birth, including the loss of a cultural and ceremonial context, especially for Indigenous women.

The family doctors who provide rural maternity care are passionate about it, and they see themselves as providing full-service maternity care, including birth and often anaesthesia. If they depart, the system radically changes. If a community loses maternity care, it tends to lose child care specialists, as well as community health workers and school health workers. Finally, although the community will be served by doctors, the kind of doctor changes. When maternity and child care are no longer in place, the doctors who serve the community are not full-service doctors. They tend to refer a lot because their skills are more limited. Unlike their predecessors, the new doctors lack a commitment to the community and don't stay long.[30]

Although these are the most extreme examples of a maternity system under stress, even women living in large urban centres are finding it increasingly difficult to find a maternity provider to attend them for their pregnancy and delivery. Why do we have a growing gap in maternity care? The answer involves multiple factors. First, the number of family physicians practising obstetrics in BC and nationally has greatly declined in recent years. Furthermore, more than twenty rural maternity services have closed in BC since 2000. Fewer family physicians are incorporating maternity care into their practices, and the age of obstetricians is increasing. This maternity care gap is even more troubling when you consider that the number of births per year in BC is projected to increase from around forty thousand to more than fifty thousand by 2020.

Although the number of posts for midwife trainees has recently increased, we are still not training enough midwives. Wait-lists at most midwifery practices are far outstripping supply. The point is not to produce just any type of care provider. The type of care midwives and many family physicians provide is exactly the type of care the great majority of the population needs—care that specifically addresses the needs of the low-risk population. The approach most of these primary care professionals employ will reduce unnecessary Caesarean sections and other procedures, while improving outcomes for mothers and babies at lower costs to the system.

In some (mostly rural) settings, collaboration between midwives and family physicians can save a maternity service from going under, avoiding a loss of culture that would make a community unattractive to young families.

If our governments truly understood that midwives provide a high level of care, with far fewer interventions, resulting in overall savings for our health care system, they would strongly promote midwifery while encouraging family physicians to take on and stay in maternity care.

Public policy decisions regarding health care, especially maternity care, need to be based not on the vagaries of a year-to-year budget cycle but on the needs of women and their families, supported by sound evidence and analysis. I've become convinced that midwives, working in innovative and collaborative models of care with other maternity care providers, are a significant part of the answer to a system under increasing stress. Midwives can increase access to maternity care in urban, rural and underserved communities and help improve health outcomes for mothers and newborns, which is why most of us involved in maternity went into this profession in the first place.

While I was chief of the department of family practice at Women's and Children's Hospitals, the position afforded me the opportunity to be a part of the British Columbia Reproductive Care Program (BCRCP). At the time, the program was occasionally asked to evaluate childbirth in particular cities or regions, because of an issue that had arisen in maternity and/or newborn care. I participated in several evaluations, always by the request of the CEO of a region. We went out as a team consisting of an obstetrician, a family physician, a maternity nurse and a midwife. We would study the situation and submit a report on our findings. Our report was detailed and contained recommendations that were not necessarily welcomed by the CEO who had requested the evaluation.

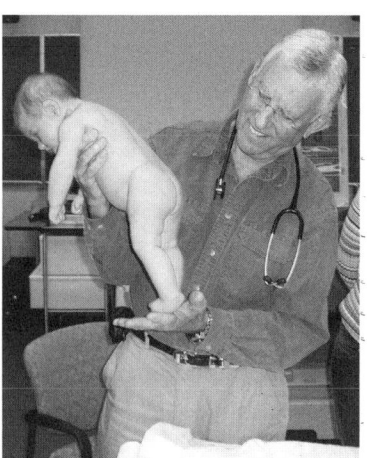

Teaching student midwives at the University of British Columbia in Vancouver.

The stimulus for one review was the threatened closure of maternity services in Nelson, BC. In this case, under pressure from the community, the CEO of the regional health authority requested the review. The CEO planned to close all services in Nelson except emergency care, thereby turning the Nelson hospital into a triage station on the way to the town of Trail. Surprisingly, the CEO committed himself in advance to follow the recommendations of the BCRCP team.

Nelson is in the Kootenays in BC's Interior, seventy kilometres from Trail, on a difficult mountainous road. It takes about an hour to ninety minutes to drive the distance, unless the road is icy and snow covered. At times, the road is impassable. Nelson was considered to have a model rural hospital. It had three general surgeons, a urologist, two internists, a pediatrician and an obstetrician, and two midwives used it as well. A large group of family physicians attended births and received backup from the obstetrician and pediatrician, and the general surgeons provided Caesarean section backup when the obstetrician was occupied or away. Moreover, it was one of the first small rural hospitals that embraced midwifery, and relations between the disciplines were outstanding.

The regional health authority was determined to close all in-patient services in Nelson, designating Trail as the regional centre—despite the dangerous route from Nelson to Trail and the fact that Nelson was also itself a de facto referral centre, draining a number of small communities in its natural catchment area. Before our review was completed and received by the CEO, he advised all the Nelson specialists to move to Trail. With the exception of the pediatrician (who was determined to stay in Nelson as a consultant to the GPs), all of the other specialists were making plans to move away from the area entirely, rather than move to Trail—some to the United States.

While one of the surgeons was making plans to leave but was still in Nelson, a Nelson resident ruptured his spleen. The surgeon operated and saved his life. There would have been no time for them to get to Trail. He would have died on the way. The health authority was unmoved.

The BCRCP recommendations were limited to birth, as was their mandate. The BCRCP strongly recommended that maternity care remain in Nelson. But the health authority did not immediately follow the recommendations. It was in this heated environment that the Nelson community and their doctors invited me to make a presentation. The meeting took place in the hockey arena. I was freezing as I stood on a thin piece of plywood placed on the ice.

The community members at first exhorted the town's doctors to take the issue to the health authority and the media. This would have taken pressure off the community members, who assumed that the doctors had the power to influence the decision. When my turn to speak came, I pointed out that the doctors would be seen as feathering their own nests and ignored. I pointed out that the only way to influence the health authority was for the community of Nelson to take direct political action and leave the docs out of it.

I suggested sitting in at their MLA's (local elected ministerial representative) office, with baby carriages and pregnant bellies. This was done. It worked for maternity care. Unfortunately, all the specialists left for parts unknown, as they said they would.

The good and bad news is that the in-patient wards vacated by the health authority's dictum, wards that were used by all types of general and specialist admissions, were now empty. The community recruited an obstetrician who would be on salary rather than fee-for-service. The obstetrician, a recent graduate from the University of Toronto, worked with the community to save maternity care in Nelson. The vacated in-patient space became a birth centre.

The health authority prohibited the obstetrician from doing major abdominal and gynecological surgical cases. Little did they know that this well-trained obstetrician could do laparoscopically what most obstetricians could only do with open surgery. Patients operated on laparoscopically get better sooner as well. The few major elective procedures went to Trail. The obstetrician has been in Nelson for more than fifteen years and has no intention of leaving, despite the fact that when a backup GP surgeon does a Caesarean section in his usual fee-for-service mode, the cost to the BC Medical Services Plan (MSP) is deducted from the obstetrician's salary.

In 2014, probably based on my work in Nelson and discussions on our maternity listserv, known as Maternity Care Discussion Group (MCDG), where I have been listmaster for more than thirty years, I was invited to assist Banff with their maternity care problem. Banff is a sweet community in Alberta well known for its skiing and other recreational activities. The little hospital in Banff was a full-service hospital mainly served by GPs, a few specialists and some GP surgeons, GP and specialty anaesthesiologists, and nurses with a range of skills. They had a maternity ward and a Level 1 nursery, capable of basic newborn care. Consultations and transfer to specialists were obtained from hospitals in Calgary, 130 kilometres away. The town of Canmore is 26 kilometres away, between Banff and Calgary on the Trans-Canada Highway. In good weather it is an easy car ride. Canmore has a small full-service community hospital, including maternity care and birth.

Banff hospital at various times has had two GPs doing maternity care and births. Now there is only one, in part because the Alberta regional health authority and the Banff hospital's CEO, in a hospital governed by a faith-based organization, actively discouraged GPs interested in birth from settling in

Banff. Hence, the single-handed GP has been the sole physician responsible for births, attending about fifty births per year, for many years. Her husband, a GP general surgeon, is available for Caesarean sections.

The community is greatly supportive of this single GP and passionate about retaining maternity care, even with low birth numbers, especially because the highway to Canmore can be snowy, slippery and dangerous. Rarely, it has been completely closed. Another unappreciated or ignored factor is that Banff hospital maternity and other services acts as an unofficial referral centre for patients from Lake Louise and other small communities as far away as the BC border. Patients travelling to Banff from these distant communities while in labour and approaching birth appreciate being able to stop in Banff rather than travelling on to Canmore.

This sole GP had superior relations with the maternity care nurses, who were devoted to birthing mothers and proud of their work, despite the small size of the service. The Caesarean section and episiotomy rates and use of other interventions in birth were very low. Outcomes for mother and baby were outstandingly good, especially compared to Canmore, where a group of GPs provided maternity care. The relatively poor outcomes in Canmore compared to Banff is especially interesting, because Canmore tends to transfer to Calgary many conditions retained by Banff, which ought to result in a lower Caesarean section rate in Canmore than Banff, but it is the opposite. One can appreciate why the Banff GP does not want to go to Canmore for her births.

The CEO of Banff hospital found that staffing the maternity service was expensive because birth timing is unpredictable. She was not impressed with the excellent results, compared to her plan for the facility. Astonishingly, what the CEO had in mind was to provide *destination plastic surgery* at Banff hospital, something the community does not need but is a big moneymaker. She advertised this service in the US, coupling the service with reduced-fee hotel accommodations in the town. Perhaps, as some joked, a ski-and-plastic-surgery package could be sold. She began promoting Banff plastic surgery in the US before she ordered the maternity service stopped, telling the sole GP to attend her births in Canmore, a decision strongly opposed by the Banff community, who knew well how excellent the maternity care and outcomes were delivered by their GP and maternity nurses.

Advertising in the US drew private-pay Americans, because plastic surgery in Banff was less expensive than comparable care in the US, and the hospital would receive US dollars to help balance its budget—with full support from the faith-based governing group in turn responsible to the Alberta regional health authority.

The plastic surgeons and anaesthesiologists, lusting after the private American dollars, fully supported the CEO and brought along a number of the other specialists to this cause. As this scenario had reached a fever pitch, I was invited to address the community, which I did after studying the many interlocking issues. Wisely, the GP attending births stayed in the background, while a variety of very sophisticated community members spoke to the issues that would affect the community. These included highway conditions, the limited bus service that was of course unresponsive to women in labour, the cost to poor and Indigenous women and families of going to Canmore, and the loss of some supports from family unable to make the trip.

It was a large and vocal meeting, with the community selling T-shirts excoriating the CEO and addressing the issues. The MLA said some waffling things and was roundly booed. He promised to look into the problem, but the community knew he would not.

I spoke to the issues I had researched, and I clearly supported the community's position. As I did in Nelson, I gave them the data to support their cause and supported the direct community action needed.

It was uplifting but useless in the end. The CEO refused to meet with the community and closed the maternity service. As the Banff hospital was closing, one patient came to the GP's clinic in active labour too late to transfer to Canmore. The GP wanted to assure the health of the fetus, so she borrowed a fetal monitor from the emergency room, with the permission of the emergency room staff. The CEO accused her of stealing hospital equipment and reported her to the hospital's Medical Advisory Committee to be sanctioned. She even involved the RCMP in an investigation. The charges never went anywhere, but still…

49. MIDWIVES AND THE HOME BIRTH DEMONSTRATION PROJECT

HOME BIRTH CAN TEACH US lots about hospital birth. As part of the introduction of midwifery in BC, in the pre-legalization or pre-regulation era, I was asked to lead a study to evaluate home births in the province. I declined, as I felt that my association with the development of midwifery was so strong that the project could be seen as a conflict of interest and therefore could endanger the results. Nevertheless, I was part of the project's design and was delighted to recommend that Dr. Patti Janssen take on the role as principal investigator. The unique design of the project allowed for a five-year study of every home birth in BC. And there were to be three comparison groups: all home births, all hospital births by the same midwives and a matched sample of physician births from the same settings for women who had the same characteristics, meaning that the women would have been eligible for a home birth, if physicians did home births, which they did not.

Another unique aspect of the study was that we did not sit around and wait for bad things to happen. A panel of experts including obstetricians, family doctors, nurses and midwives would review every transfer and every potentially problematic outcome so that a report could be sent to the BC

College of Midwives, which could then issue directives to correct problems before they became serious.

The results of the study were startling to some.[31] The outcomes for the newborns were similar for the three groups. However, midwives at home had the best outcomes in terms of much lower use of procedures, based on intention to treat, meaning that once labour began at home, the outcome was assigned to the home birth category, not to the hospital. Otherwise, the hospital might be credited with outcomes that belonged with the home birth analysis. Interestingly, the planned hospital births by the very same midwives had more in common with physician births in hospital than with their own births at home, illustrating the pernicious effect of the hospital environment.

The results of the study, and two related ones from Ontario, demonstrated the safety of home birth when midwifery is regulated and conducted by university-educated midwives who are fully integrated into a health care system, which accepts the midwives as valuable partners.

Despite the studies' clearly demonstrated safety of home birth, a substantial number of practitioners and members of the public cannot accept that home birth could be as safe as hospital birth, where all the needed bells and whistles are ready at hand, this despite the fact that midwives are fully and repeatedly trained in maternal and newborn emergencies, and they carry oxygen and other emergency supplies to every home birth. Of course I have never said that home birth is safe in all situations. In BC and Ontario, where midwives are university educated and home birth is regulated and fully integrated into the birth system, it is safe.

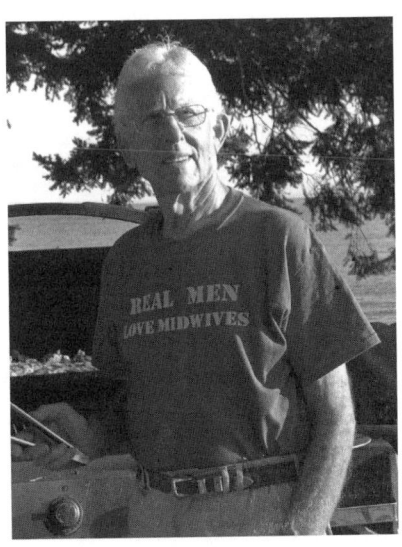

Real men love midwives.

The same positive result might not occur in situations where the system is not there to support the midwives. In the US, in settings where midwives are unsupported or where the conventional medical system is hostile to home birth, we can hardly expect that home birth is as safe as it is in Canada or in certain European settings.

Canadian obstetricians' mostly negative attitudes toward home birth are based on lack of experience with "ordinary" home birth or collaboration with midwives. Each discipline operates in its own silo. Medical practitioners tend to remember only the cases sent to hospital for problems, even though the most common problem is the need for additional pain relief that is not available at home, like epidurals. Furthermore, medical practitioners can all remember particular cases where rapid response to either maternal or newborn emergencies saved the day. How could such emergencies be anything other than worse off at home?

Home birth is not intrinsically safe. Hospital birth is also not intrinsically safe. It depends. It depends on the individual setting and the individual skills of the practitioners. If home birth is as safe as the BC and Ontario studies indicate, when it seems like hospital birth ought to be safer, then something has to be going on in the hospital to cause problems that are avoided at home. It is a case of apples and oranges. In the home, the comfortable setting and intimacy of midwifery care prevent some problems that are actually *caused* by the hospital environment. In contrast, there are undeniably some rare problems that can occur at home that might be better managed in the hospital. These two systems of care each have their issues, but they are *not the same issues.* Even though these different environmental issues balance out in the raw numbers of maternal and newborn outcomes, showing an equivalency of maternal-newborn outcomes in hospital and at home, in the two settings the risks and benefits are different, as are the complications and protections. How do you quantify the benefits of intimacy in the home versus availability of immediate backup in the hospital? Or how do you quantify the effect of overuse and misuse of technology in the hospital versus the potentially protective effect of being in the home. Mistakes can occur in both settings, but they are different mistakes. In summary, if we could make the hospital as comfortable as home, who would not want to give birth in hospital? But we can't, so informed women will select the type of provider that fits their needs and values.

50. BIRTH ROOMS AND DOULAS COME TO VANCOUVER

IN AN ATTEMPT TO IMPROVE the atmosphere of birth and gain the benefits of both birth rooms and the presence of doulas at birth, BC Women's established an environment to support both.

I had been part of developing the birth room and the investigator of a study of the birth room at the Jewish General, so I was familiar with the model.[32] As in many places across the country, hospitals were moving away from having labour in one room, warehousing babies in a large nursery (without rooming-in) and accommodating the mother for recovery in yet another room. "Musical maternal beds" were certainly going out of favour. In Vancouver, we were aware of the new trend and changed part of the hospital to single-room maternity care on the second floor, away from the operating rooms. A single nurse looked after the mother during her labour and birth, and she also looked after the newborn and mother in the same room until discharge.

As with any new development, there was resistance. We worked hard to encourage acceptance of the idea of single-room maternity care. The pediatricians and anaesthesiologists were initially skeptical or even against it. Some claimed that the time from the elevators on the second floor to the operating rooms on the first floor was too long. I pointed out that we were talking about five to seven minutes, whereas there were many places in BC where it was thirty minutes to hours for a Caesarean section—nevertheless with good outcomes. Eventually, the staff accepted, even liked, the concept.[33]

I will never forget a birth room experience in which a young Indigenous woman was labouring with her first birth. There were twelve people in the room, family and friends supporting her. As one was massaging the labouring mother, another was massaging the massager, and so on down the line. There was singing and chanting. When the labouring woman was finally too exhausted to carry on and the baby was not descending, I called for an anaesthesiologist to administer an epidural. The anaesthesiologist who arrived was a stand-in (locum), a man unfamiliar with such "nonsense." "Everyone out. I cannot do my work with people looking over my shoulder," he said. I negotiated to get down from twelve to six family members. The epidural was administered. The patient slept, woke up and birthed her baby. The selective use of epidurals is the way to go.

During my more than ten-year tenure as chief of the family practice department at BC Women's and Children's, a series of related issues evolved. The midwife development was big, but in parallel, the doula movement was developing throughout North America and eventually reached the hospital. Doulas are not responsible for the birth. The doctor or midwife is professionally responsible. The doula's role is only to support the mother and not interfere with the health provider. I supported the doula movement from its start and have been on the board of Doulas of North America (DONA).

As the doula phenomenon evolved, it was not surprising that there was resistance from some quarters. Some obstetricians felt that doulas were usurping the role of the obstetrician. Even some nurses and midwives thought the same. Few providers had read the literature on the positive effect of doulas on key maternal and newborn outcomes. Some questioned the relevance for the typical North American environment, as almost all of the early doula studies took place in the developing world or inner-city settings.

As the doula movement reached the hospital floor, it became clear that all doulas were not the same. Why wouldn't we expect that to be the case, as we know that all doctors or nurses are not the same? With trainees, I wrote about this issue and the conflicts that can occur when well-intentioned doulas run up against providers that the doulas know are not practising in an evidence-based way.[34] These conflicts also emerged from our national study of the attitudes and beliefs of all caregivers. As well, it is clear that many women do not appreciate the potential importance of the doula role.[35]

Kathie Lindstrom was in charge of doula education at Douglas College. It was her role to train and monitor doulas in BC, but there are also other, less well-known doula organizations. It is even possible for a non-certified midwife in BC to avoid being arrested for practising midwifery without a licence by calling herself a doula, but that is another story.

Kathie and I put together a doula course for first-year medical, nursing and midwifery students. They learned interdisciplinary care and came to appreciate the other trainees' skill sets. Although it was an elective course, it had an important positive effect on overall medical student training. When a doula-trained medical student reached their third-year OB/GYN clerkship, they already knew a great deal about normal birth. Typically, student clerks were encouraged to concentrate on births where there were problems, thereby creating a distorted view of birth. They spent lots of time assisting at Caesareans or complex instrumental births. But our doula-trained med students insisted on having a normal birth experience and some of their classmates saw their example and came to realize the importance of doulas and normal birth.

The doula model was then extended to a special ward for substance-using women. Again, medical, nursing and midwifery students took responsibility for the women and helped in the birth. The women often gave up drugs and kept their babies. Previously, the usual approach was to apprehend the baby. The woman would then repeat the process and come to the hospital again pregnant and drug-dependent. Dr. Ron Abrahams and members of the BC Women's Family Practice Maternity Service deserve credit for changing a practice that was wrong and dangerous.

51. INTERNATIONAL COOPERATION: IT'S NOT ALL ABOUT BIRTH

EARLY ONE MORNING IN 2001, while I was recovering from an all-night labour and birth, I received an urgent phone call from a dear colleague in Haifa, Israel.

Shmuel said, "Michael, I have a problem. I just received a panicky phone call from Tanya, the girlfriend of a young man whom I have cared for since childhood. Both she and Jan had recently been discharged from the army and were travelling the world. They are in Vancouver, where they attended a walk-in clinic because Jan had a high fever. He was told it was flu and to go and rest in the hotel. It does not sound like flu to me!"

Two hours later, Jan appeared, extremely pale, sweating and leaning heavily on Tanya, looking like he was about to fall over. On physical exam, this powerful ex-paratrooper had a weak and rapid pulse, and his liver and spleen were enlarged. Heart failure was clear. It was extraordinary that he could even walk. I arranged some urgent blood work, which showed profound anemia and a white blood cell count of 186,000, almost all immature white cells. Diagnosis: acute (myelogenous) leukemia.

I called the hematology-oncology ward at Vancouver General Hospital (VGH), which rapidly sent an ambulance. Then, with remarkable international cooperation, the head of service at the hematology-oncology ward called his counterpart at the Technion's hospital in Haifa, and together they planned the treatment.

Blood and platelet transfusions began, followed quickly by chemotherapy. But as the chemo quickly destroyed the abnormal white cells, the broken-down cancer cells were thrown at his liver and kidneys for processing. His kidneys shut down and dialysis was started to compensate. He developed pulmonary edema, fluid in the lungs, and went on a respirator.

About that time, his mother arrived from Israel. I was soon visiting with the entire family, first in the ICU and later in a cubicle on the hematology-oncology ward. The young couple was amazing. We did our best to make the mother welcome, and soon Jan's father arrived.

The recovery was striking. In a few days, it was hard to imagine how very sick Jan had been. After a couple of weeks, he was ready to return to Israel, where he received an autologous (his own) bone marrow transplant and made a full recovery. Within a few months, we received an invitation to the wedding. But after much discussion, Bonnie and I felt we could not attend. We knew that we were going to miss a wonderful event. We had developed such a close relationship with the family, who saw us as saving their son's life and playing a central role in the fact that there was a marriage at all. Why not go?

The problem was the Second Intifada. Before this Palestinian uprising in the early 2000s, and the harsh reprisals by the Israeli government and military, I had extensive and cordial relationships with many Israeli family medicine colleagues who were at the forefront of peace activities, treating patients in Arab and Bedouin villages and helping train Palestinian physicians. After the Intifada, almost all of my Israeli physician friends changed. Most dropped their peace work and took the position that the Israeli government was justified in their actions. This change, combined with the unrelenting and uncritical support for the Israeli government and its military's treatment of the Palestinians, supported by both the American and Canadian Jewish Congresses, fractured my relationships. I stopped working with my Israeli colleagues, but I deeply missed those relationships.

I did not see how Bonnie and I could feel comfortable at the wedding, given we were so against the response from the Israeli government and many of our friends. It probably was the wrong decision, one that was not repaired for many years, not until Bonnie and I went on a Compassionate Listening tour of Israel and the Palestinian West Bank in 2008.

Despite the horror of the wall the Israeli government built to separate Israel and the West Bank, we came to appreciate both sides of the conflict by listening, without judging, to the stories of parents on both sides who had lost children and family. This is basic family medicine. We do not judge. One of the principles of compassionate listening is that your enemy is someone whose story you have not heard. On that tour, we met Israelis and Palestinians and really learned to listen to all sides. We asked lots of questions but did not engage in arguments. As Elie Wiesel said, "Questions unite people, answers divide them." This tour allowed me to think more clearly about my Israeli physician friends and finally visit with them and renew our friendship. There was a parallel with some of the conflict between obstetricians and family doctors. The techniques of compassionate listening help there as well. We also got to visit with Jan and his parents, their family now including two kids.

About two weeks after Jan returned to Israel, I got a call from a family physician up the Fraser Valley that demonstrated the adaptability of family practice. I knew the doctor from one of the Advanced Life Support in Obstetrics courses that I ran. "Michael, I have a problem. I have a patient who is due tomorrow but I can't care for her. Her husband has been admitted to Vancouver General Hospital with a lymphoma. She won't leave his side. Can you take over and attend her birth?"

And so later that afternoon I met a charming young woman about to have her first baby. On exam she was perfectly well. Her GP had sent her records, so I had the full picture. The next morning, she went into labour and quickly delivered an eight-pound girl, without any pain medications and with no tears or any other birth trauma. Then she asked for immediate discharge so that she could join her husband, so at six hours, I discharged her. Next day I made a "home visit" at VGH, where she was calmly nursing her baby in her husband's isolation room—the very same room vacated by Jan, the Israeli ex-paratrooper. Her husband had Burkitt's Lymphoma. He had a full course of treatment and has done very well, as have mother and baby. Something special about that room?

52. LIVING WITH A DIAGNOSIS: MORE SYSTEM FAILURES

I WONDER SOMETIMES IF I somehow attract professional complexity and role confusion. Certainly, that was a major feature of the care surrounding Bonnie's dramatic illness and recovery. I am afraid that it is more likely that this issue arises all the time—only others may feel too intimidated by the system to interact or even intervene. I wish that many other caregivers could experience compassionate listening. Learning to put your professional self into the shoes of family members ought to be part of the medical curriculum. As with Bonnie's care, in the care of my father I would have dearly loved to sit back and be a grateful family member—but stuff kept happening.

My father, Philip, at almost eighty-four years old, had a rocky recovery from multiple coronary bypass surgery. He was discharged to our Vancouver apartment on drugs to deal with the intermittent heart failure he experienced in hospital.

After a week, he was well enough to return to his home a ferry ride away on the Sunshine Coast, where he and my mom had recently moved. I went to see him on the weekend and found him again in heart failure. I arranged an urgent visit with his family doctor. Later that week, I was so concerned about how my dad sounded over the phone that I cancelled my office hours and grabbed the ferry, finding him worse than ever. His family doctor and I agreed that he needed hospitalization back in the tertiary care centre in Vancouver.

After a few days in hospital, my father was again discharged to our Vancouver apartment, a scant few hours off a dopamine (a major drug) and furosemide drip. Bed crunch, I was told.

He stayed three days at our Vancouver home, and I was forced into an unwanted role as physician because his doctor was a ferry ride away on the Sunshine Coast. I juggled medications, trying to balance low-cardiac output confirmed by low blood pressure and concurrent signs of congestive heart failure. I was getting very anxious.

I omitted one dose of his prescribed powerful diuretic because I was worried about his very low/undetectable blood pressure and about the possibility of low-output cardiac failure. The diuretic could have led to circulatory collapse. I returned home a few hours later to find my dad in peripheral shutdown, with blue nail beds and almost no air entry in the right lung and obvious dullness in the other lung.

I brought my father to the emergency room, where I met a junior resident who listened respectfully and carefully to my history, asked appropriate clarifying questions, and then did his own complete and accurate exam. He reported to the head of the emergency room, who acted with both medical and humane effectiveness, acknowledging my distress and understanding fully how difficult it was for me to play the role that had been thrust upon me. This is the way it ought to be. The medical resident on the coronary care service, however, stated that if I had not omitted the diuretic my father might not now be in the emergency room.

This punitive nonsense felt very familiar, both from my experience with Bonnie's care and my role as family physician, often sending a patient to a tertiary care centre for assessment or treatment, only to have a smart-assed resident who neither knows the patient nor the circumstances, pontificate about what the proper treatment should have been or question the need for the referral. This kind of arrogance is unfortunately much too common. As director of outreach for a tertiary care centre, the persistent complaint I heard from rural GPs was about the behaviour that I had just experienced, in which the receiving institution or physician, lacking adequate appreciation of the realities of rural practice, puts down the referring physician for not doing one thing or another or missing a diagnosis that turned out to be the correct one all along.

During rounds in the coronary care unit several days later, that same resident, clearly uncomfortable with my presence, and wondering out loud if she should say in my presence what she was about to say, inquired if we had reached the end of our therapeutic approaches in an eighty-three-year-old man with obviously compromised ventricular function.

It was not so obvious to me, and certainly not clear to my dad's own cardiologist, that we had reached the end of the line, or that we even knew what was going on. The resident indicated that it was time to consider "dying with dignity." I indicated that I was in favour of dying with dignity at the right time, but at the moment I preferred "living with a diagnosis," as it was unclear why my father was in this state.

The coverage system changed at the beginning of a new week. My father was now under the care of a second ICU cardiac care team. The attending physician found my few questions irritating and made it clear that he was busy and I was taking up too much of his time.

However, the nursing care was superb, technically and personally. The nursing staff genuinely cared about my dad, my mom and me. My dad was improving, so he was moved to the adjacent step down unit. The care was good but the nurses harried. My father was rapidly moved to a medical ward where care could be managed by his own cardiologist. To protect myself from assuming the role of physician for my father, I arranged for my own Vancouver family doctor to be my father's GP, standing in for his GP on the Sunshine Coast.

The transfer to the medical ward was accomplished. However, although the idea of the transfer was good, the timing was not. It occurred very late in the day. When I arrived at about 9 p.m., I found my dad had been situated in the back of a large ward at the most remote location from the nursing station—not a good idea for a still unstable patient.

My dad was disoriented and delusional. His nail beds were blue, and he was on oxygen, his respirations laboured. Blood pressure was low. On my brief, superficial and clandestine exam, I found that again he had evidence of heart failure. His right lung field was dull and he was coughing and wheezing slightly. I did not have a stethoscope, which was just as well, as this would probably have been pushing the limits of the son role, the stethoscope being the symbol of physician power and control.

The coughing and wheezing were a new finding. I communicated my concern to the nurses, who appropriately responded by phoning the medical resident on call. A new and harried resident was at first cordial. I politely and cautiously told her of my observations and findings. It was clear that she was uncomfortable with me in this role. She tried in not very subtle ways to assert her dominance. I wondered if we were caring for my father or engaging in power politics.

Since it was late in the day and the resident was preoccupied with a large number of other patients, I offered to encapsulate the complex history (the chart was inches thick) to save her time and proposed to show her some relevant information in the chart, information that my dad's cardiologist and GP had shared with me. The resident became irate, stating flatly that it was inappropriate for me to look in the chart (which I had not done), and that I was inappropriately involved in my father's care. She kept talking about how old my dad was, implying directly and indirectly that I was being unrealistic in my expectations. I had not expressed any expectations. I knew how sick my dad was, that he might die anytime. But I wanted high-quality, appropriate care for the present crisis, many aspects of which were new.

To counter ageist thinking and to give the resident the flavour of the person my dad was and how well he was just a relatively short time ago, I explained that less than a year ago, at the age of eighty-two, he had packed up the house that he and I had built over ten years of summers and weekends and drove with my mother four thousand kilometres across the US and Canada to their new country home on the Sunshine Coast.

Her response floored me. "If it were up to me, I would take away the driver's licences of all those old people. They have no peripheral vision and their reflexes are bad. I am afraid whenever I see one of them on the road." I was so stunned that I was mute. The resident wrote some orders and left without reading the chart. Competent physicians always look at the big picture. They gather information from as many sources as they can, and then make the necessary decisions on their treatment. Physicians who behave the way that I witnessed are insecure in their own competence.

Meanwhile, the nurses tried to gain control of the total ward situation. They were appropriately worried about my dad's location and confusion, and concerned about his falling out of bed, so they asked me how I would feel about their placing him in restraints. I did not doubt their staffing situation and the reality of my father's disorientation. I told them to do what they needed to do, and I helped them set it up.

Sometime in the night, the nurses, knowing well the delicate situation, had moved my dad up to a room adjacent to the nursing station. By the following day, having gotten appropriate support from her attending physician, the offending resident started the required dopamine drip, which stabilized the situation. My father was no longer in peripheral shutdown. His blood pressure was up and confusion was gone, though he was still a very sick man.

However, the following day, the nursing coverage was limited and my father was again very unstable. He was returned to the original cardiac ICU, where nursing, resident and attending staff struggled to understand a situation that should have been improving but was not. A new attending cardiologist covering for the weekend acknowledged his inability to sort out the problem, discussed his difficulties openly with me and the resident, and arrived at a plan to obtain the needed information to form the basis of therapeutic interventions. Since I had been respectfully included in the complex discussions but clear that the responsible physician was in charge, I was able to relax and stay in the role of concerned family member.

The same medical resident who had inappropriately criticized me for omitting the diuretic dose at home now openly discussed her concerns and frustrations. Perhaps the resident was less tired and harassed; perhaps the resident had followed a behavioural cue from the very caring attending cardiologist. Physicians-in-training are often like chameleons—taking on the characteristics of their teacher role models. A week later, when yet a new cardiac attending physician arrived to take over, he also discussed his confusion with me, his belief that the main problem was pulmonary, not cardiac—the lungs, not the heart. All cardiac meds were stopped while vigorous pulmonary treatments were carried out, with good results. There had been no need for any conflict around me and my father's care. All that was required was open discussion of the concerns of a family member who happened to be a physician.

In a couple of days, my dad was no longer an "interesting patient," and no longer in need of ICU care. Discussions began again about sending him to a ward. But the attending cardiologist was responsive to my concerns about limited and overworked nursing and medical support, and open to my suggestion that rapid transfer to his own community GP might be the best plan.

I had gotten to know many of the GPs on the Coast because of what our family called a Friday night special. Typically, I took the ferry from Vancouver to the Coast every Friday night to find my dad in cardiac failure. I would then have to bring him to the emergency room at the small community hospital and spend the weekend watching while the medical staff got him out of heart failure.

The community GPs took turns staffing the emergency room and simultaneously covered the hospitalized patients at the small hospital, including the two-bed ICU. This is typical for small Canadian rural communities. Over many Friday night specials, I had gotten to know and respect a large number of the covering GPs.

One night soon after my father was discharged back to his home on the Sunshine Coast, where he would be followed by his own GP, he was once again the victim of a Friday night special, this time so serious that he was occupying one of the two beds in the little ICU. It was midnight and my dad was being cared for by yet another new GP, Dr. Ron Estey. My dad was again in low-output cardiac failure. He was in a low oxygen state with blue nail beds and mental confusion.

Dr. Estey and I were talking at the bedside about what to do. It was a conversation between two colleagues, one in charge and the other a physician-son. Sharing the complexities, we both knew that he needed dopamine, a powerful drug requiring careful monitoring. The nurse covering many sick patients throughout the hospital allowed that she could not manage dopamine, given her other multiple responsibilities. She said that hospital protocol required that if my dad needed dopamine, he would have to be transferred back to Vancouver. In his confused state, my dad nevertheless overheard enough of the conversations to say he would rather die than go back to Vancouver. We understood.

Dr. Estey decided that he would manage the dopamine himself, and by about 4 a.m. my father's nail beds were pink and he was resting peacefully. Both of us were feeling comfortable with each other. I explained with embarrassment that I felt it necessary to change doctors. Not your problem, Dr. Estey replied. "By the way," Dr. Estey said, "you have a terrible memory."

I said, "About what?"

He responded, "You don't remember me! When I was one of a group of medical students at McGill, where you were the chief resident in the newborn ICU at the Royal Victoria Hospital, we spent six weeks with you and you looked after us well. It will be my pleasure to care for your father."

With my father's permission, I arranged for my former student to take over his care, and my mom's as well. The GP was clearly in charge, but he saw me as a collaborator. I tried not to abuse his openness but felt comfortable discussing my concerns. And he easily agreed to see my dad on Wednesdays. The Friday night specials disappeared.

Dr. Estey determined that one of my dad's medications might have been contributing to increased pulmonary vascular resistance and discontinued it. My dad improved dramatically. Home oxygen was stopped and medications reduced. Things were looking good, but we knew it was going to be a long haul.

Once again, my father's care, as was the case with Bonnie's care, illustrated the importance of being engaged with the staff and being vigilant. That does not mean getting in the way, but stuff happens. If you are not a physician, you still need to remain vigilant and express your thoughts. If something does not seem right, it probably isn't.

My dad lived a much diminished but happy life for another three years. His medical problems were difficult, complex but manageable. He died at home in his sleep.

Advocacy for my dad or other family members has been critical, but self-advocacy is also important, physician or not. Just before leaving Montreal, I experienced a fascinating event at the very hospital where I was head of family practice and well known to the nursing staff, with whom I had cordial relationships. I thought I was done struggling with control issues. Guess not. I had developed a kidney stone that became lodged in the wall of the bladder and would not pass. I had surgery by an excellent urologist. Not surprisingly, there was lots of post-operative bleeding, and I assumed I had blood clots in my bladder and bladder outlet, as I could not pass urine. Lying in my hospital bed, I became more and more distressed as my bladder increased in size. In fact, I palpated my bladder as elevated to the level of my belly button. I thought I must have a couple of litres of urine. No wonder I was distressed.

I rang the bell for the nurse, informing her that I was obstructed and needed the surgeon. The nurse said, "Dr. Klein, don't be such a baby. I don't want to bother the surgeon for nothing." When the nurse left, I quietly went into the utility room to get a catheter and catheterized myself for about two litres of bloody urine with lots of clots. In my backless hospital gown, I walked to the nursing station and presented the nurse with a bedpan of the stuff. She called the surgeon, who resolved the problem. On the topic of physicians receiving the best or worst care, it was a painful lesson in how to be a pain in the ass—or in this case, the bladder.

53. MY MOTHER'S DEATH

I WAS AT WORK IN Vancouver. Mid-morning I got a call from my eighty-five-year-old mother, Annie, on the Sunshine Coast. She sounded very unwell. I dropped everything and grabbed the ferry to the Coast. When I arrived at her home, an elderly friend was with her. It was clear to me that she was very sick, but it was not clear from what. I called her GP, Dr. Ron Estey, who advised that I keep in touch with him. He would make a house call after his clinic was over, but I should take her to the emergency room at any time if I was concerned.

We made her some soup and Jell-O, and she began to look and sound better. The friend left, so I was alone with my mom while she slept. After a couple of hours, she asked me to help her to the bathroom. On route to the bathroom, she suddenly collapsed. She was pale and without a pulse.

Fortunately, I had immediate access to a speakerphone and thus was able to dial 911 and talk with the operator while carrying out full CPR, including cardiac massage and mouth-to-mouth ventilation on the floor where she had collapsed. The ambulance team arrived in about fifteen minutes, during which time there had been no positive results from my efforts.

The ambulance technicians were prepared to initiate defibrillation and continue resuscitation efforts, but they accepted my request that we stop everything. It was obvious to me that further efforts would fail and be disrespectful to my mother. What happened next is dictated by protocol. The emergency team is required to notify the RCMP when an unexpected death occurs. So within the next hour, a young RCMP officer arrived, assessed what he thought to be the situation, asked me a few irrelevant questions and then began to stretch yellow crime tape around my mother, who was still lying on the floor where she had collapsed.

Notably absent from his inquiry was a history of my mother's multiple cardiac and other chronic illnesses. What the hell? He was accusing me of killing my mother. It was so macabre that I could not take it seriously. Bonnie and Seth were on their way from Vancouver, but I was alone. In fact, the behaviour of the RCMP officer was so inappropriate and the scene so bizarre that in a strange way it was helping me with my grief.

I called Dr. Estey, who said he would come as soon as his clinic was over. I called my neighbour Dr. Russ Kellett, the only obstetrician on the Coast, who lived just down the street. Russ arrived in good time and the two of us sat around the kitchen table drinking beer, while the great detective continued stretching yellow tape around the crime scene and taking photographs.

Soon the RCMP officer's superior arrived in his curling shoes. He had been called from his time off to do the investigation. The two of them continued their process, the superior also failing to ask the appropriate questions. Russ and I chatted away, vaguely aware of the evolving and wildly inappropriate crime scene.

Next to arrive was the coroner. In the small town of Gibsons, the coroner is also the funeral director, and I knew him from our positive interaction around my father's death. He was the first to make a clear statement to the RCMP: "What the hell are you doing? Don't you know that this elderly woman has been very sick for many years? Haven't you got something better to do?"

No response from the cops, who continued their investigation of the great crime. I allowed to Russ that I was reminded again of Arlo Guthrie's song "Alice's Restaurant," in which a small-town cop takes many colour, glossy eight-by-ten photographs of the crime of littering.

The next to arrive was Dr. Estey. He was less charitable than the coroner. "What the hell are you doing, you morons?" he expostulated, while making threatening gestures toward the cops. "Get the hell out of here. Did you bother to ask anything about the health of Mrs. Klein?" He finally managed to convince the cops to take down their yellow tape and leave.

The next day, I received a phone call from the young RCMP officer, who claimed to need some further information for his files. I hung up on him. A few weeks later, I learned that the young officer had been transferred to another jurisdiction. It seemed that his inappropriate behaviour had been a frequent occurrence. It did not explain the actions of his superior officer, who remained in the community.

Nothing further ever developed. We had a lovely multi-generational memorial for my mom in a local restaurant, attended by many friends and family. It was more like a wake, with singing and live music. In the seven years that she had lived on the Coast, in her mid-eighties, my mother had developed friendships with a large circle of women her age with whom she attended exercise classes, swimming classes, and a spinners and weavers guild. As well, a surprising number of young people had seen her as a surrogate grandmother and also attended the memorial. I got to play "Shalom Aleichem" on my clarinet and then, with local musician friends, some klezmer tunes while the neighbourhood danced. The RCMP was not invited.

54. MORE ADVOCACY: BUTTING IN WHERE YOU HAVE NO BUSINESS

ONE LATE WINTER IN VANCOUVER, I learned that the son of one of my staff members had had a serious accident and was at VGH. He was a student at Simon Fraser University and had been on a winter field trip. Somehow, he had fallen hundreds of feet down an icy slope and spent most of the day alone at the bottom of a ravine. Ultimately, he was rescued by helicopter and taken to VGH, where he arrived with a temperature of thirty-four degrees Celsius, unconscious and unresponsive. He was in the ICU with an enormously swollen head and on a respirator.

My staff member told me that the ICU and neurosurgical staff had been trying unsuccessfully for days to wean him off the respirator. I learned that there was talk of turning off the respirator, which would lead to the patient's death. I asked about the role of the family GP and was told that he had refused to come to the hospital, where he felt unwelcome. I asked if there had been a family conference. No, there had not.

With my staff member's enthusiastic approval, being neither a family member nor a treating physician, I visited the ICU. The patient was deliberately paralyzed so that he could be ventilated. I learned from the nurses that the patient's pupils were reactive. There was no evidence that he was brain dead. It was just a question of somehow getting him off the respirator.

I contacted my neurosurgeon friends at Children's to see if they could offer anything. They found the story strange but were unwilling to involve themselves in another colleague's territory. I then contacted Bonnie's neurosurgeon, Dr. Skip Peerless, in London, Ontario. He had spent many years in Vancouver and was well respected. He faxed me a detailed protocol for weaning such patients off the respirator.

Armed with the Peerless protocol, I arranged a family conference at the ICU. It was most awkward. Who the hell was I? The neurosurgeons were hostile. What right had I to interfere? Then, to make matters worse, I presented them with the Peerless weaning protocol.

It worked. Long story short, the patient graduated with honours from Simon Fraser University. I admit this is an extreme example. The message again is that if the situation feels wrong, it often is, and physician or not, family member or not, advocacy and common sense demand that you intervene. We all know that mistakes happen, and they happen often. Trust your instincts and act on them. Advocacy is not a crime.

55. NOTHING FAILS LIKE SUCCESS

It seemed like my experiences in Mexico and Ethiopia were in a sense following me even in Vancouver. During a major epidemic of measles in Vancouver and the Lower Mainland, I reflected on how the success of modern immunization has set the stage for vaccine deniers and the rise of diseases that were thought to have disappeared from modern societies. Measles, whooping cough and a series of other preventable diseases are reappearing. The issue of parental autonomy versus the safety of the community is vigorously debated. In some communities the issue turns around freedom of choice, whereas in others entry to school cannot happen without demonstrated immunization records. Those vigorously opposed to this directive are choosing home schooling. My experiences in Mexico and Ethiopia and even Montreal showed the consequences of an unimmunized population and led me to think deeply about how inappropriately relaxed we have become about protection from preventable diseases.

Measles is a disease that today's Western communities have not experienced. They may think of it as a simple rash. No problem. Just live with it. I remember well, in the pre-immunization days, getting measles myself. I had to stay in a dark room because of the pronounced light sensitivity. I was miserable, with a high fever, coughing and choking. In fact, the rash is the least of it. It is an infection of the breathing tubes, including bronchopneumonia, general aches and pains, high fever and, in the worse cases, serious inflammation of the brain, or encephalitis. And, by the way, a rash.

In the winter of 2015, in both the US and Canada, an outbreak of measles was underway, setting loose what seemed like an endless discussion about routine immunization. On one side were spokespeople for public health, shocked that routine immunization should be up for debate. On the other side were impassioned individuals and some organized anti-immunization crusaders, for whom no scientific argument was permissible.

In Canada, some calling themselves naturopaths were claiming that they had products that could replace immunization and prevent measles and other diseases that are prevented by routine childhood immunization. These bogus products are attractive to those who distrust conventional medicine. On the CBC, I heard a discussion that pitted public health officials against a woman who claimed that she had done her research, which showed that serious adverse events were common in routine immunization. What she called research was actually online chats that she had with other people who were against immunization. She also brought up as "evidence" the long ago discredited research that falsely claimed a link between measles and autism.

When the interviewer pointed out that her choice not to immunize her children was reducing herd immunity and thereby putting others, including immune-compromised children and adults, at risk of preventable diseases, she replied that she was sorry about that. When the interviewer pointed out that the source of recent outbreaks were certain religious communities and other groups that were against immunization, she replied that they had a right to their beliefs and that in the end it was about "freedom of choice."

Shortly thereafter, I heard stories on the CBC claiming adverse events following immunization of girls for HPV, the virus that causes cervical cancer. These stories included an amazing array of events that could hardly be associated with anything, including drowning in a bathtub. The stories all had in common the inability of the storytellers to appreciate the difference between *association* and *causation*.

Why the debate? Immunization campaigns of the past have been so successful that the public does not have personal experience with the diseases that have been prevented, including diphtheria, whooping cough, tetanus, polio, meningitis and ear infections caused by *H. influenzae.* In the very recent past it was usual for the public to have had direct experience with these diseases. For example, the public knew of President Franklin Delano Roosevelt's much-diminished state after he had polio. It is remarkable to think that FDR was so weakened that if he had died a little earlier from the disease, World War II might have been lost.

I also have personal experience of these diseases, beginning at six months of age, when I had a severe case of whooping cough. My family camped on the beach, exposure to salt air all that could be offered. And I'll never forget spending a week in a dark room with measles.

Even my mother suffered from shingles and the related post-herpetic neuralgia, which made her last years painful from a disease now preventable by immunization. Shingles can be a life-altering disease for the elderly, occurring as our immunity and defences naturally decline. Shingles is caused by the same virus that gave us chicken pox, or varicella, in childhood. We don't have to get it. As elders now, Bonnie and I have received the varicella-zoster vaccine.

The recent epidemic of mumps in professional hockey players reflects waning immunity. It's no joke, as some of those young men will have become infertile as a result, not to mention the joys of painful testicles.

The very success of immunizations has allowed those who deny their efficacy or have issues with modern medicine to find a receptive audience. These deniers distrust doctors and science, sometimes with good reason. They allow their own personal "freedom" to do what they please with their bodies to trump the public good.

Of course, vaccine side effects do occur, but their frequency is many orders of magnitude less than the frequency of major complications and death from the diseases they prevent. Unless we reach those who distrust modern approaches to disease prevention, diseases that were eliminated are at risk of reappearing. The earth is not flat. The climate is warming. Vaccines work and have eliminated diseases that we hope never to see again.

56. PRIVATE FOR-PROFIT CARE

I HAVE HAD A PERSPECTIVE on the funding and organization of medical care that is unusual, as I practised in Canada before universal health care (during my residency), in Rochester without universal health care and back in Canada with a single-payer national health care system. Fundamental to remaining in Canada was my need to practise in a universal health care system. This issue has come to the fore recently because of a 2016–18 case at the British Columbia Supreme Court, in which the owner of a private clinic, Dr. Brian Day, took BC to court over his belief in his right to charge whatever he likes for his services, even those already covered by the public purse. This followed a provincial audit of his clinic, where the auditors found that in one three-month period he had overbilled or double-billed the province almost half a million dollars. In a sense, the Supreme Court case brought by the owner of the private clinic can be seen as a countersuit.

Dr. Day claimed that people should have the right to jump the waiting list by using their own funds. The cure is worse than the disease. What is not appreciated is that if we were to follow Dr. Day's prescription for reducing wait times in the public system, we would be at risk of losing our unique Canadian health care system altogether, as privatization undermines the need-based equity and fairness that characterize our system. Somehow, some well-to-do Canadians in a position to influence the way our system functions have promoted the idea that market forces in health are an appropriate way to solve some of our system's real problems. Those who cannot afford private care may be told by their surgeon that they must somehow come up with the funds for his private care or suffer irremediable damage while waiting in the public system. For a desperate and vulnerable patient, this form of blackmail is unethical.

Led by physicians who stand to gain from being able to overcharge and double-bill patients for services (mainly surgical) that are already covered by our Medicare system, some Canadians have come to believe that it is reasonable to buy your way to the head of the line. The promoters of privatization are promulgating the myth that letting some patients jump the queue actually shortens the line for those who cannot afford to pay. Although this might be true if we had an infinite number of doctors and nurses, that is not the case. Our resources are limited; hence, queue jumpers actually lengthen the line for the rest of us. And our Canadian sense of fairness and equity that defines us, our collective commitment to our social safety net, is being destroyed.

Promoters of private solutions often claim that there are unemployed surgeons who would not go private if health authorities would open and staff more operating rooms. Although there are a few, mostly orthopaedic, surgeons who cannot get hospital privileges because of scarce operating rooms, there are reasons for this. There are open surgical positions outside of the main population centres that would love to have an orthopaedic surgeon—but the surgeons don't go there. And many older surgeons resist retirement, which would make room for younger surgeons. Some health authorities, however, do indeed restrict operating room time as a means of balancing their fixed budgets, or they contract out surgical care to private facilities under the public purse rather than open operating rooms in public hospitals.

As the public ages and demand inevitably increases for services like hip, knee and eye surgeries, our politicians and the public need to decide to allocate more funds for this need. It is a political choice to spend more for needed services, like opening operating rooms, that will lead to shortened wait-lists. Fortunately, as of this writing, the BC government has injected substantial dollars into opening operating rooms to shorten waiting lists for hip and knee surgery and other surgical procedures.

Our health care system has not had a major overhaul since its inception in the 1970s, but we need to work on fixing the problems through comprehensive health care reform, without destroying a system that most Canadians feel is an expression of the highest values in our society. Those who see an increase in private care as the main way to fix the system seem unable to separate their own financial benefit from the needs of the nation.

Although I looked in the US for a warm place to live and work where Bonnie could be independent, in the end I was so distressed by the US private for-profit system that permeated everything from how poor people were cared for to the educational system, I felt I had no choice but to remain in Canada.

It is useful to think about how Bonnie was flown without charge from Quebec to Ontario on a specialized intensive care jet to receive landmark surgery unavailable in Quebec, how her many months in hospital cost as much as renting the room TV. Or when I required back treatments then unavailable in Canada, Quebec paid for me to receive care in Minneapolis. Unlike what many in the US believe, there are no restrictions in Canada on choice of physician, assuming availability. In fact, our system is largely entrepreneurial and uncontrolled, unless the doctor is on salary, which is still rare. Some would say that ours is not a health care system at all but a system of paying doctors and hospitals for providing services according to a schedule of payments. And we are unique among comparable Western societies because we do not fund essential drug costs for the patient.

In Canada, as health authorities see or even encourage the private system as a means of taking pressure off strained budgets, motivation to fix or improve the public system is reduced. This problem is exacerbated because it is the wealthier and more powerful in society who can afford private care. As these "movers and shakers" leave the public system, leadership with the commitment to improve the system for everybody is lost.

We have undergone a vicious cycle of neglect of the public sphere, which has been allowed to deteriorate. However, multiple studies in and outside Canada have shown that central control of the wait-list, rather than leaving it to individual surgeons, can dramatically reduce waiting times. Moreover, the needs of patients on the list change all the time. Evaluation and re-evaluation of patients on the list needs to take place by the patients' family doctors and specialists working together—so that those who need to be at the top of the list get there, while others who may not need to be on the list for surgery at all can be removed. The demand for overused MRIs also needs to be managed centrally, as many on the wait-list don't need to be there and would be better served by less expensive laboratory tests. Privatization is not the answer—improving the existing system is.

I am astonished, though I ought not be, that Americans, who are one disease short of being destitute, believe that single-payer health care is bad for them. The US population refuses to embrace the obvious in part because they've been scared with terms like "socialism" and the spectre of a Canadian system where they claim falsely that people cannot choose their own doctor and will not receive the care that they need. Of course Canadians can see their own doctor, as many times as they need, without cost to them, just by showing their Medicare card. US private insurance interests willfully propagate lies about the Canadian health care system, and a naive and unsophisticated American public believes ignorant legislators in the pocket of lobbyists.

For Bonnie and me, this degradation of the Canadian public health system is particularly difficult to witness. Having returned to Canada, and remained in Canada, to avoid the worst of US financially driven medicine, it is especially hard to watch our country inexorably move in the very direction that we sought to avoid.

So if care on either side of the border is so different, why are procedure rates in maternity care so similar? Although procedure rates are somewhat higher in the US, one would expect there to be a much larger difference based on the vastly different way that health care is funded and organized. Caesarean section rates make the point, with rates in Canada hovering at or slightly above 25 per cent, whereas in the US it is more like 30 per cent, with pockets in the US up to 50 to 60 per cent and in Canada around 40 per cent. How can this be? This relative lack of difference between the US and Canada in maternal procedure rates happens because the *training* of physicians on both sides of the border is so similar that it overwhelms system differences. Most doctors in Canada, like in the US, operate on a fee-for-service basis. Their motivation is similar. Doctors in both countries are independent contractors who are largely in control of their practice, though both are subjected to increasing regulation and controls.

In Canada, there are only a few examples—in Quebec and Ontario—where physicians are on salary. In British Columbia, this is exceedingly rare. This model of payment is seen more often in rural and remote settings, where it is called alternative payments. The effect of this model is that the physicians and the rest of the health care team consider their patient to be a member of the community that they serve. In these cases, all on salary—doctors, nurses, nurse practitioners, public health nurses and the other members of the health care team—meet regularly to figure out what to do. In this setting, creative solutions are found: group prenatal care, group cardiac and hypertension care, home visits and more. Innovation not only happens, but it is necessary. So-called physician extenders like nurse practitioners can be fostered because not only do the doctors not have to pay for them out of pocket, but they can also focus on collaboration and using the full skill set of all providers.

57. WINDING DOWN

MY LAST OFFICIAL ACADEMIC ROLE as a member of the UBC Department of Family Practice began in early 2000, when I was appointed to head up the Clinical Scholars Program, a post that I held for seven years. I was responsible for providing support and training to practising family physicians who had an important research idea that they wanted to pursue. Even late in my academic career, the job was one of the most satisfying. We took in about four trainees per year. Their research ideas came directly from their practice. We provided a stipend so that they could afford to take time out of their practice to do the research. Then we provided mentorship to make their idea come to life. Many of the studies were published, and some of the trainees went on to become academic family physicians and conductors of important primary care research.

One of my last trainees was Lynn Farrales. Lynn practised family medicine in an area where many immigrants lived. Her project was to have been a study of problems in that community. Then the unimaginable happened. Just as Lynn was about to start the clinical scholar training, she and her husband, John, had an unexplained and unforeseeable stillbirth at the very end of her normal pregnancy. She delivered a perfectly formed little girl, Scarlett Amelia, who had died for no apparent reason. She called me to share the terrible news and requested a leave of absence of a year, planning to enter the program with the following group. After a long discussion about what she was experiencing, I agreed to her request.

After some early follow-up phone calls, I called Lynn again, four months after the event, proposing that she consider changing her topic to stillbirth and rejoining the program. There was and is much to still learn about this condition, how to prevent it and how to cope with such an event. I tried to persuade Lynn gently that, as awful as her experience was, she was positioned to make an important contribution. She agreed, first returning to the program part time and then full time.

Lynn has done nationally funded primary research on stillbirth, has founded a self-help organization for parents who have experienced stillbirth and is presenting a series of papers for publication on the subject. Lynn and John are waiting to be adoptive parents.

In part, what made me so interested in Lynn pursuing this line of stillbirth research was the parallel with my own path. My best research has always come directly from my personal or practice experience. Trying to answer questions that materialize from practice is the driver for the most important contributions.

In 2018, as I reach the end of my active research career, I find that the most useful thing I can do is spend my time supporting younger colleagues as they work on new ways to provide accurate and user-friendly information to the new generation of women as they approach their first births. I love working with enthusiastic midwives and family physicians as they train to provide women-centred care. This is how I ought to be spending my time.

It is hard to watch the way that birth has been transformed into a technological experience without trying to do something about it. We know that providing intimate care and information to women leads to the best outcomes. We know that providing high-risk care to high-risk women improves care, but the provision of high-risk care to low-risk women makes them sick.

Another factor that can set the stage for a redesign of the maternity care system stems from new epidemiologic data that shows, for the first time in North America, maternal mortality rates are rising, and there is a suggestion, too, that newborn complications are also on the rise. In BC, the provincial medical officer labelled this increase in serious maternal health outcomes a public health issue. Against this backdrop, obstetricians are aging and fewer family doctors are deciding to provide maternity care. Older maternity nurses with the needed skills to support women who do not have an epidural are retiring. As we train insufficient numbers of midwives and maternity-committed family doctors, the system is on the road to collapse. This might be the right time to engage in a total system redesign.

To rebuild the system, ministries of health and education will need to collaborate in the design of a maternity care system that will produce the correct number and correct types of birth providers. Midwives will be the centre of the primary care maternity system, collaborating with devoted family doctors who are committed to the field. Doulas will also be key to a rational system, since research demonstrates how doulas improve outcomes for mothers and babies. Obstetricians, rather than competing for patients, will be trained to provide consultation and appropriate medical and surgical support to the primary care providers.

Such a rational system will lead to a major reduction in Caesarean sections and other procedures, optimal outcomes for mother and baby, and a dramatic reduction in hospital admissions and length of stay. Such a rational system built through the training of fewer obstetricians and more midwives and family physicians, and through the inevitable requirement for fewer maternity nurses and expensive maternity beds, will lead to major savings that can be passed on to the health authorities for better use.

AFTERWORD

WHEN I WAS EDUCATED AT Stanford I was not exposed to family practice, so it took me a number of years to discover it and recognize the benefits of the approach. Throughout my practice and in my personal life I encountered the need to advocate for the patient and the family. The system often makes unintended mistakes. We all know this, so it is necessary for doctors and family alike to be vigilant and intervene if necessary. No one knows the patient better than the family. The integration of the family into medical care is not a conflict but leads to enhanced care. Skilled physicians know this and are comfortable integrating the observations of family members into the care, whereas insecure physicians may find this threatening.

Good medical care involves thinking about the patient in the context of their life. Creative integration and experimentation with a variety of modalities—such as alternative therapies—will lead to the best outcomes. I often struggled to have this approach considered as part of care, as such "soft" and "unscientific" approaches are out of the experience of many conventional medical practitioners. I learned very early in training and practice, and in the care of Bonnie, that doctors need to be modest in what they believe about their contribution to cure.

I realize that my experiences in Ethiopia and Mexico were unusual and life altering—rare for medical students caught in the rigid structure of usual medical training. I was fortunate to have a medical school dean who was flexible enough to allow me the time to follow my passion. These experiences made me a better doctor and provided me with skills that most students never develop. More of this kind of flexibility in medical education is needed.

Now that I no longer see patients clinically, I remain engaged in medical issues and continue to teach research methodology to family practice residents, and clinical and research skills to midwifery students.

It was hard for me to stop seeing patients in my family practice—especially maternity care, my central area of passion, but in the end, I found that I was concerned about maintaining the quality of my practice. In my late sixties, I found the long sleepless nights increasingly difficult. It took me many days to recover from an all-nighter. My experience reflects the natural fraying at the edges that all older doctors experience—but I miss it.

Continuing as the listmaster of the Maternity Care Discussion Group (MCDG) helps keep me current. It is the only multidisciplinary maternity discussion group worldwide and a unique forum for obstetricians, family physicians, maternity nurses, midwives and doulas to share clinical experiences and solve problems—even political problems. Such a self-help discussion group is a model of non-territorial inter-professional cooperation. To join the list, contact me at mklein@mail.ubc.ca.

Maternity care is under stress around the world as medicalization of childbirth continues to accelerate, while society and professionals alike increasingly see childbirth as just an opportunity for things to go wrong. Fortunately, there are movements in the other direction. Women are driving this movement, insisting that the control of childbirth remain in the hands of the women having babies.

This is the current version of the earlier movement to "humanize" childbirth by getting partners into the delivery room and limiting unnecessary procedures. The movement toward normal physiological childbirth, though historically necessary, cannot easily go against current trends, but determined consumers are having an impact in some settings. Although midwives provide excellent one-to-one clinical care, they will also need to enter the political arena, with their natural allies, to maximize their impact on overall maternal health.

Increasing the midwifery resources to be able to care for appropriate low-risk women for birth in hospital and at home, and increasing the number of family doctors who include birth in their practice, will result in the need for fewer obstetricians. The obstetricians will then provide only the complex care needed for selected patients on referral from midwives and family doctors.

To rationalize maternity care, ministries of health and ministries of education will need to plan together how many of what type of provider will be required—and who will train them and where they will be trained. This is a tall order but becoming more possible as the system fails and women are finding it increasingly difficult to obtain the right care from their chosen provider. The pressure to plan for the future will become more and more clear, and serious discussions about how to care for pregnant women will have to take place at the highest governmental levels.

This evolving process also finds resonance among those who are paying the bills, including insurance companies, health authorities and even national health care schemes. The time may be right for a major change in how maternity care is provided, but it will take an enormous commitment from many players to realize what is best for childbearing women. If successful, the paradigm of childbirth as a disease may shift to a view of childbirth as a transformative, growth-promoting and joyous happening.

The earlier portion of my career and practice involved many areas, including public health and international health. So why did I focus so heavily on maternity care? For me, it was a natural evolution. My rather backward path from being a pediatrician/neonatologist to a family physician allowed me to see this area of care from several perspectives. My unique training and experience allowed me to operate at the interface of pediatrics, newborn intensive care, obstetrics, nursing, midwifery and family practice. Here, I felt I would make my greatest contribution in practice, training and research.

Maternity care, however, provides a window on the values of a society, just as, in a bizarre way, episiotomy provided a vehicle to traverse and understand a complex birth system. What do we feel is important as a society? How do we think about the future of society, the role of women, the value of children? Although I moved more and more from a general family practice to one focused mainly on birth, I nevertheless stayed committed to seeing birth in the context of society.

When birth is seen primarily as an expensive, unpredictable and dangerous event, birth and those who provide birth care will be sidelined. Hospitals and health authorities will download the care of pregnant women to large centralized hospitals where well-meaning strangers will do their best to care for women they do not know. This dystopic picture is well underway, while some attempts to slow or stop the trend are also happening. How this struggle will resolve remains to be seen.

Although I still engage with maternity care at several levels, it is time to focus more on children and grandchildren and the outdoors, and worry more about the planet and the world that we are leaving for them.

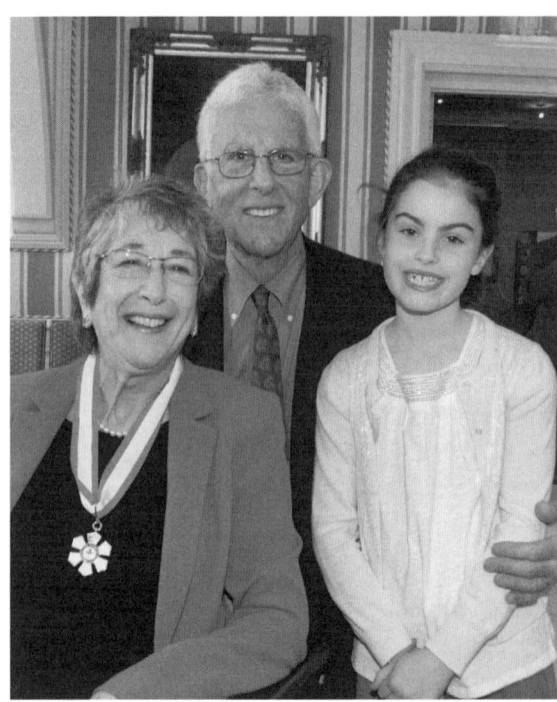

With our granddaughter, Zoe, as Bonnie was inducted as an officer of the Order of Canada.

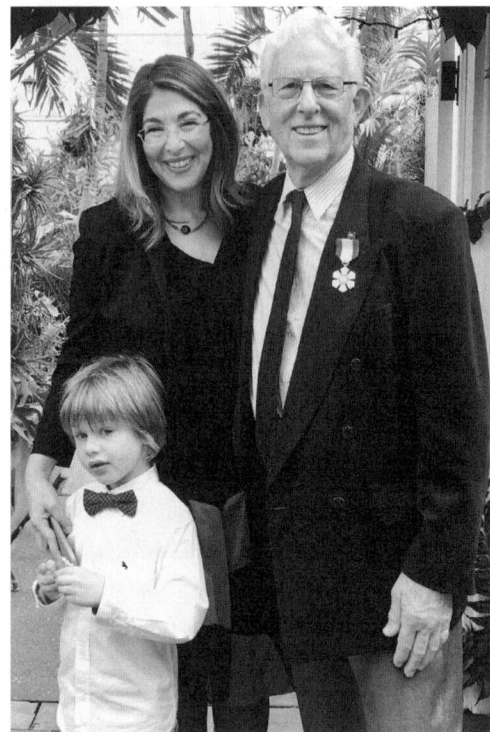

Me after receiving the Order of Canada, with my daughter, Naomi, and her son Toma.

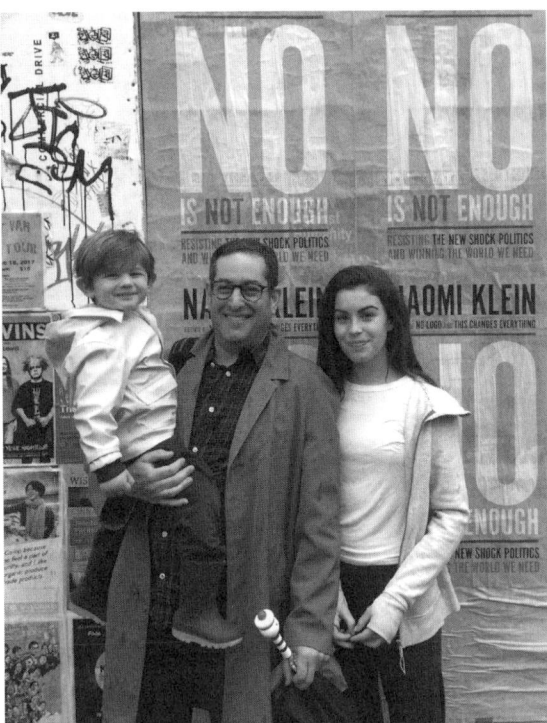

Aaron (age 3), Seth
and Zoe (age 13)
at an anti-pipeline
demonstration in 2017.

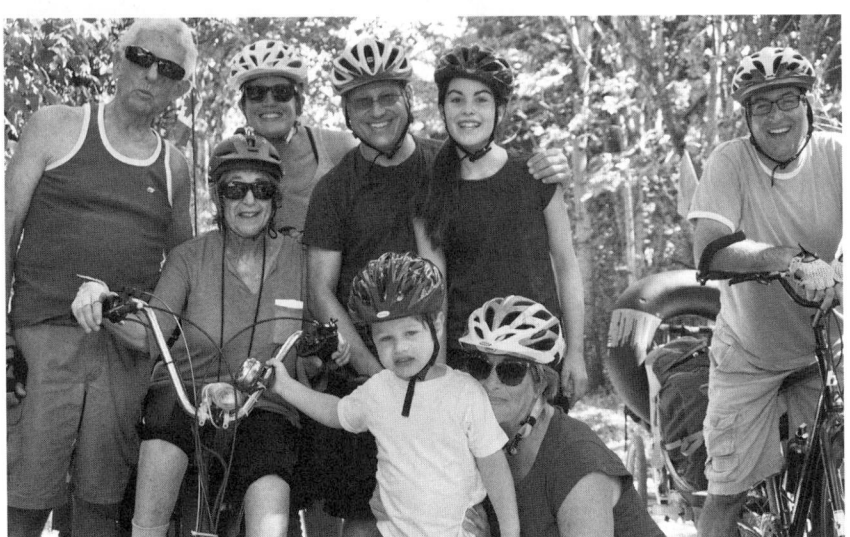

The whole family during a bike trip. Back row, left to right: me, Christine
Boyle (Seth's wife), Avi Lewis (Naomi's husband), Zoe, Seth (on bike).
Front row, left to right: Bonnie, Toma (Naomi and Avi's son), Naomi.
Baby Aaron (son of Seth and Christine) is asleep in the carrier.

FINAL REFLECTION: MY MENTORS

ONE OF THE CHALLENGES OF writing this book has been to find the "through-line" from the resilience of the human body and spirit to birth in practice and as a metaphor, my struggles with the US Army, Bonnie's illness and recovery, the role of midwives and family physicians in fixing the health care system, the need to protect the Canadian health care system from privatization, the intersection of attitudes and education, and how advocacy is critical to successful caring—all supporting the overall theme. The patients' stories have been chosen to reflect these issues.

As I put the final touches on the manuscript, I was struck by another linkage to the overall narrative: my mentors. Who were they? Why was I attracted to them and what was our shared experience? Starting with my first mentor, Robert Greenberg, to Louis Fraad, Marshall Klaus, Robert Usher, Eugene Farley, Sheila Kitzinger, Murray Enkin—each one was both a leader in their field and one who contested conventional wisdom. They all share the title: dissident doctor, challenging the medical status quo.

ENDNOTES

1   Saroj Saigal, "Quality of Life of Former Premature Infants during Adolescence and Beyond," *Early Human Development*, Volume 89, Issue 4 (April 2013): 209–13.

2   Kara Stanley, *Fallen: A Trauma, a Marriage, and the Transformative Power of Music* (Vancouver: Greystone Books, 2015).

3   Michael C. Klein, et al., "Earthenware Containers As a Source of Fatal Lead Poisoning— Case Study and Public-Health Considerations," *New England Journal of Medicine*, Volume 283, Issue 13 (September 4, 1970): 669–72.

4   Michael C. Klein and Leo Stern, "Low Birth Weight and the Battered Child Syndrome," *American Journal of Diseases of Children*, 122 (1971): 15–18.

5   Michael C. Klein, Diana Elbourne, Ivor Lloyd, "Booking for Maternity Care: A Comparison of Two Systems," *Journal of the Royal College of General Practitioners*, 31 (April 1985): 1–17.

6   Michael C. Klein, "Contracting for Trust in Family Practice Obstetrics," *Canadian Family Physician*, 29 (1985): 2225–27.

7   Ruta Westreich, et al., "The Influence of Birth Setting on the Father's Behavior toward His Partner and Infant," *Birth*, Volume 18, Issue 4 (December 1991): 198–202.

8   Joseph B. DeLee, "The Prophylactic Forceps Operation," *American Journal of Obstetrics and Gynecology*, 1 (1920): 34–44.

9   Thomas Kuhn, *The Structure of Scientific Revolutions* (Chicago: University of Chicago Press, 1962).

10 Joseph B. DeLee, "The Prophylactic Forceps Operation," *American Journal of Obstetrics and Gynecology*, 1 (1920): 34–44.

11 Ibid.

12 Michael C. Klein, "Studying Episiotomy: When Beliefs Conflict with Science," *Journal of Family Practice*, Volume 41, Issue 5 (November 1995): 483–88.

13 Michael C. Klein, et al., "Relationship of Episiotomy to Perineal Trauma and Morbidity, Sexual Dysfunction, and Pelvic Floor Relaxation," *American Journal of Obstetrics and Gynecology*, Volume 171, Issue 3 (1994): 591–98.

14 Michael C. Klein, et al., "Physician Beliefs and Behaviour within a Randomized Controlled Trial of Episiotomy: Consequences for Women under Their Care," *Canadian Medical Association Journal*, Volume 153, Issue 6 (September 15, 1995): 769–79; and Michael C. Klein, et al., "Determinants of Vaginal/Perineal Integrity and Pelvic Floor Functioning in Childbirth," *American Journal of Obstetrics and Gynecology*, 176 (February 1997): 403–10.

15 Bonnie Sherr Klein, *Slow Dance: A Story of Stroke, Love and Disability* (Toronto: Knopf Canada, 1997).

16   Bonnie Sherr Klein, *Shameless: The Art of Disability* (National Film Board of Canada, 2006).

17   Michael C. Klein, "Too Close for Comfort? A Family Physician Questions Whether Medical Professionals Should Be Excluded from Their Loved Ones' Care," *Canadian Medical Association Journal*, Volume 156, Issue 1 (January 1997): 53–55.

18   Chiara Saroli-Palumbo, et al., "Pre-University Students' Attitudes and Beliefs about Childbirth," *Canadian Journal of Midwifery Research and Practice*, Volume 11, Issue 2 (Summer 2012): 27–37.

19   Michael C. Klein, "Quick Fix Culture: The Caesarean-Section-on-Demand Debate," guest editorial, *Birth*, Volume 32, Issue 3 (2005): 161–4; and Michael C. Klein, "Obstetrician's Fear of Birth: How Did It Happen?" *Birth*, Volume 32, Issue 3 (2005): 207–8.

20   Michael C. Klein, et al., "Epidural Analgesia Use As a Marker for Physician Approach to Birth: Implications for Maternal and Newborn Outcomes," *Birth*, Volume 28, Issue 4 (2001): 243–48.

21   Michael C. Klein, et al., "Does Delivery Volume of Family Physicians Predict Maternal and Newborn Outcome?" *Canadian Medical Association Journal*, Volume 166, Issue 10 (2002): 1257–64.

22   Michael C. Klein, "Cesarean Section on Maternal Request: A Societal and Professional Failure and a Symptom of a Much Larger Problem," *Birth*, Volume 39, Issue 4 (December 2012): 305–10.

23   Michael C. Klein, et al., "Epidural Analgesia Use As a Marker for Physician Approach to Birth: Implications for Maternal and Newborn Outcomes," *Birth*, Volume 28, Issue 4 (2001): 243–48.

24   Patti Janssen, Michael C. Klein, and J.H. Soolsma, "Differences in Institutional Cesarean Delivery Rates: The Role of Pain Management," *Journal of Family Practice*, Volume 50, Issue 3 (March 2001): 217–23.

25   Michael C. Klein, "Epidural Analgesia: Does It or Doesn't It?" *Birth*, Volume 33, Issue 1 (2006): 74–76.

26   Michael C. Klein, et al., "The Attitudes of Canadian Maternity Care Practitioners towards Labour and Birth: Many Differences but Important Similarities," *Journal of Obstetrics and Gynaecology Canada*, Volume 31, Issue 9 (2009): 827–40; and Michael C. Klein, et al., "Attitudes of the New Generation of Canadian Obstetricians: How Do They Differ from Their Predecessors?" *Birth*, Volume 38, Issue 2 (2011): 129–39.

27   Michael C. Klein, et al., "Family Physicians Who Provide Intrapartum Care and Those Who Do Not: Very Different Ways of Viewing Childbirth," *Canadian Family Physician*, Volume 57, Issue 4 (2011): 139–47.

28   Michael C. Klein, et al., "Birth Technology and Maternal Roles in Birth: Knowledge and Attitudes of Canadian Women Approaching Childbirth for the First Time," *Journal of Obstetrics and Gynaecology Canada*, Volume 33, Issue 6 (2011): 598–608.

29   Michael C. Klein, et al., "Mothers, Babies and Communities. Centralizing Maternity Care Exposes Mothers and Babies to Complications and Endangers Community Sustainability," *Canadian Family Physician*, Volume 48 (July 2002): 1177–79.

30   Christine Miewald, et al., "You Don't Know What You've Got Till Its Gone: The Role of Maternity Care in Community Sustainability," *Canadian Journal of Rural Medicine*, Volume 16, Issue 1 (2011): 7–12.

31   Patti Janssen, et al., "Outcomes of Planned Home Birth with Registered Midwife versus Planned Hospital Birth with Midwife or Physician," *Canadian Medical Association Journal*, Volume 181, Issues 6–7 (September 15, 2009): 377–83; erratum in *CMAJ*, Volume 181, Issue 9 (October 27, 2009): 617.

32   Ruta Westreich, et al., "The Influence of Birth Setting on the Father's Behavior toward His Partner and Infant," *Birth*, Volume 18, Issue 4 (December 1991): 198–202.

33   Sue Harris, et al., "Single Room Maternity Care: Perinatal Outcomes, Economic Costs, and Physician Preferences," *Journal of Obstetrics and Gynaecology Canada*, Volume 26, Issue 4 (2004): 33–40.

34   Sabha Eftekhary, Michael C. Klein, and Shi Yi Xu, "The Life of a Canadian Doula: Successes, Confusion, and Conflict," *Journal of Obstetrics and Gynaecology Canada*, Volume 32, Issue 7 (2010): 642–49; and Natalie Lea Amram, et al., "How Birth Doulas Help Clients Adapt to Changes in Circumstances, Clinical Care, and Client Preferences During Labor," *Journal of Perinatal Education*, Volume 23, Issue 2 (Spring 2014) 96–103.

35   Michael C. Klein, et al., "Birth Technology and Maternal Roles in Birth: Knowledge and Attitudes of Canadian Women Approaching Childbirth for the First Time," *Journal of Obstetrics and Gynaecology Canada*, Volume 33, Issue 6 (2011): 598–608.

ACKNOWLEDGMENTS

To Bonnie Klein, Seth Klein, Naomi Klein, Henry Klein, Andreas Schroeder, Kara Stanley, Louise Dennys and Dr. Danielle Martin for providing detailed reading of an earlier version and offering most helpful comments. To Dave Roche, who urged me to read sections of the book publicly. To Duncan Etches, my GP and friend, and long-time friend and colleague Dr. Vania Jiménez, for encouraging me to write this book. To Carol Herbert, who not only provided important editorial comments but, most of all, as head of family practice at UBC, gave Bonnie and me the needed opportunity to relocate to Vancouver. To Dr. Demissie Habte, who was my mentor in Ethiopia, and my other mentors: Drs. Robert Greenberg, Marshall Klaus, Eugene Farley and Murray Enkin, all of whom were accessible and showed me the right path. Robert Usher, mentor and dear friend, taught me neonatology and how to argue strongly without animosity. To McGill dean Richard Cruess, who had faith and bailed me out when I ran out of funds for the episiotomy trial. To Janusz Kaczorowski, my long-time research collaborator, whose research and educational skills made it all possible. To Diana Elbourne, Iain Chalmers and Sir Alec Turnbull, who mentored me while I was on sabbatical in Oxford and helped me develop my research trajectory. To Drs. Cheryl Levitt, Michael Dworkind and the other doctors at Herzl, who cared for me and did my patient care work when Bonnie was severely ill. To nurses Karen Tafler and Barbara North, who as nurse practitioners made it possible for me to run the department at the Jewish General Hospital/Herzl Family Practice Centre with an almost full practice. They too pitched in when Bonnie was ill. With great gratitude to my editor, Amanda Lewis, who helped me shape the book from a disconnected series of stories to one that I hope has internal coherence.

BIBLIOGRAPHY

Amram, Natalie Lea, Michael C. Klein, Heidi Mok, Penny Simkin, Kathie Lindstrom, and Jalana Grant. "How Birth Doulas Help Clients Adapt to Changes in Circumstances, Clinical Care, and Client Preferences During Labor." *Journal of Perinatal Education*, Volume 23, Issue 2 (Spring 2014) 96–103.

DeLee, Joseph B. "The Prophylactic Forceps Operation." *American Journal of Obstetrics and Gynecology*, 1 (1920): 34–44.

Eftekhary, Sabha, Michael C. Klein, and Shi Yi Xu. "The Life of a Canadian Doula: Successes, Confusion, and Conflict." *Journal of Obstetrics and Gynaecology Canada*, Volume 32, Issue 7 (2010): 642–49.

Harris, Sue, Malcolm D. Farren, Patti Janssen, Michael C. Klein, and Shoo K. Lee. "Single Room Maternity Care: Perinatal Outcomes, Economic Costs, and Physician Preferences." *Journal of Obstetrics and Gynaecology Canada*, Volume 26, Issue 4 (2004): 33–40.

Janssen, Patti, Michael C. Klein, and J.H. Soolsma. "Differences in Institutional Cesarean Delivery Rates: The Role of Pain Management." *Journal of Family Practice*, Volume 50, Issue 3 (March 2001): 217–23.

Janssen, Patti, Lee Saxell, Lesley A. Page, Michael C. Klein, Robert Liston, and Soo K. Lee. "Outcomes of Planned Home Birth with Registered Midwife versus Planned Hospital Birth with Midwife or Physician." *Canadian Medical Association Journal*, Volume 181, Issues 6–7 (September 15, 2009): 377–83; erratum in *CMAJ*, Volume 181, Issue 9 (October 27, 2009): 617.

Klein, Bonnie Sherr. *Slow Dance: A Story of Stroke, Love and Disability*. Toronto: Knopf Canada, 1997.

———. *Shameless: The Art of Disability*. National Film Board of Canada, 2006.

Klein, Michael C. "Cesarean Section on Maternal Request: A Societal and Professional Failure and a Symptom of a Much Larger Problem." *Birth*, Volume 39, Issue 4 (December 2012): 305–10.

———. "Contracting for Trust in Family Practice Obstetrics." *Canadian Family Physician*, 29 (1985): 2225–27.

———. "Epidural Analgesia: Does It or Doesn't It?" *Birth*, Volume 33, Issue 1 (2006): 74–76.

———. "Nothing Fails Like Success—The Great Immunization Debate." *Birth*, Volume 42, Issue 2 (June 2015): 97–99.

———. "Obstetrician's Fear of Birth: How Did It Happen?" *Birth*, Volume 32, Issue 3 (2005): 207–8.

———. "Quick Fix Culture: The Caesarean-Section-on-Demand Debate." Guest editorial. *Birth*, Volume 32, Issue 3 (2005): 161–4.

————. "Studying Episiotomy: When Beliefs Conflict with Science." *Journal of Family Practice*, Volume 41, Issue 5 (November 1995): 483–88.

————. "Too Close for Comfort? A Family Physician Questions Whether Medical Professionals Should Be Excluded from Their Loved Ones' Care." *Canadian Medical Association Journal*, Volume 156, Issue 1 (January 1997): 53–55.

Klein, Michael C., Diana Elbourne, and Ivor Lloyd. "Booking for Maternity Care: A Comparison of Two Systems." *Journal of the Royal College of General Practitioners*, 31 (April 1985): 1–17.

Klein, Michael C., Robert J. Gauthier, James M. Robbins, Janusz Kaczorowski, Sally H. Jorgensen, Eliane D. Franco, Barbara Johnson, Kathy Waghorn, Morrie M. Gelfand, Melvin S. Guralnick, et al. "Relationship of Episiotomy to Perineal Trauma and Morbidity, Sexual Dysfunction, and Pelvic Floor Relaxation." *American Journal of Obstetrics and Gynecology*, Volume 171, Issue 3 (1994): 591–98.

Klein, Michael C., Stefan Grzybowski, Sue Harris, Robert Liston, Andrea Spence, Grace Le, Dorothea Brummendorf, Sharon Kim, and Janusz Kaczorowski. "Epidural Analgesia Use As a Marker for Physician Approach to Birth: Implications for Maternal and Newborn Outcomes." *Birth*, Volume 28, Issue 4 (2001):243–48.

Klein, Michael C., Patti Janssen, Laurie MacWilliam, Janusz Kaczorowski, and Barbara Johnson. "Determinants of Vaginal/Perineal Integrity and Pelvic Floor Functioning in Childbirth." *American Journal of Obstetrics and Gynecology*, 176 (February 1997): 403–10.

Klein, Michael C., Stuart Johnston, Jan Christilaw, and Elaine Carty. "Mothers, Babies and Communities. Centralizing Maternity Care Exposes Mothers and Babies to Complications and Endangers Community Sustainability." *Canadian Family Physician*, Volume 48 (July 2002): 1177–79.

Klein, Michael C., Janusz Kaczorowski, James M. Robbins, Robert J. Gauthier, Sally H. Jorgensen, and Arvind K. Joshi. "Physician Beliefs and Behaviour within a Randomized Controlled Trial of Episiotomy: Consequences for Women under Their Care." *Canadian Medical Association Journal*, Volume 153, Issue 6 (September 15, 1995): 769–79.

Klein, Michael C., Janusz Kaczorowski, Jocelyn Tomkinson, Nazli Baradaran, Rollin Brant, and the Maternity Care Research Group. "Family Physicians Who Provide Intrapartum Care and Those Who Do Not: Very Different Ways of Viewing Childbirth." *Canadian Family Physician*, Volume 57, Issue 4 (2011): 139–47.

Klein, Michael C., Janusz Kaczorowski, Jocelyn Tomkinson, Nazli Baradaran, Rollin Brant, Jalana Grant, Sharon Dore, Anne Brasset-Latulippe, and William Fraser. "Birth Technology and Maternal Roles in Birth: Knowledge and Attitudes of Canadian Women Approaching Childbirth for the First Time." *Journal of Obstetrics and Gynaecology Canada*, Volume 33, Issue 6 (2011): 598–608.

Klein, Michael C., Janusz Kaczorowski, Jocelyn Tomkinson, Nazli Baradaran, Wendy A. Hall, William Fraser, Robert Liston, Sabha Eftekhary, Rollin Brant, Louise C. Mâsse, Jessica Rosinski, Azar Mehrabadi, Sharon Dore, Patricia C. McNiven, Lee Saxell, Kathie Lindstrom, Jalana Grant, and Aoife Chamberlaine. "The Attitudes of Canadian Maternity Care Practitioners towards Labour and Birth: Many Differences but Important Similarities." *Journal of Obstetrics and Gynaecology Canada*, Volume 31, Issue 9 (2009): 827–40.

Klein, Michael C., Robert Liston, William Fraser, Nazli Baradaran, Jocelyn Tomkinson, Janusz Kaczorowski, Rollin Brant, and the Maternity Care Research Group. "Attitudes of the New Generation of Canadian Obstetricians: How Do They Differ from Their Predecessors?" *Birth*, Volume 38, Issue 2 (2011): 129–39.

Klein, Michael C., Rosalie Namer, Eleanor Harpur, and Richard Corbin. "Earthenware Containers As a Source of Fatal Lead Poisoning—Case Study and Public-Health Considerations." *New England Journal of Medicine*, Volume 283, Issue 13 (September 4, 1970): 669–72.

Klein, Michael C., Andrea Spence, Janusz Kaczorowski, Ann Kelly, and Stefan Grzybowski. "Does Delivery Volume of Family Physicians Predict Maternal and Newborn Outcome?" *Canadian Medical Association Journal*, Volume 166, Issue 10 (2002): 1257–64.

Klein, Michael C., and Leo Stern. "Low Birth Weight and the Battered Child Syndrome." *American Journal of Diseases of Children*, 122 (1971): 15–18.

Kuhn, Thomas. *The Structure of Scientific Revolutions*. Chicago: University of Chicago Press, 1962.

Miewald, Christine, Michael C. Klein, Catherine Ulrich, David Butcher, Sabha Eftekhary, Jessica Rosinski, and Andrea Procyk. "You Don't Know What You've Got Till Its Gone: The Role of Maternity Care in Community Sustainability." *Canadian Journal of Rural Medicine*, Volume 16, Issue 1 (2011): 7–12.

Saigal, Saroj. "Quality of Life of Former Premature Infants during Adolescence and Beyond." *Early Human Development*, Volume 89, Issue 4 (April 2013): 209–13.

Saroli-Palumbo, Chiara, Ray Hsu, Jocelyn Maffin, and Michael C. Klein. "Pre-University Students' Attitudes and Beliefs about Childbirth." *Canadian Journal of Midwifery Research and Practice*, Volume 11, Issue 2 (Summer 2012): 27–37.

Stanley, Kara. *Fallen: A Trauma, a Marriage, and the Transformative Power of Music*. Vancouver: Greystone Books, 2015.

Westreich, Ruta, Liliane SpectorDunsky, Michael C. Klein, Apostolos Papageorgiou, M. Kramer, Morrie M. Gelfand. "The Influence of Birth Setting on the Father's Behavior toward His Partner and Infant." *Birth*, Volume 18, Issue 4 (December 1991): 198–202.

INDEX